P R A I S E   F O R

MODERN DAY HOUDINI

"What a treat to be taken 'backstage' into a profession
that has fascinated people since Harry Houdini.
A behind the scenes of the world's greatest escape artist.
An incredible read about the planning, pain, motivation,
endurance, and fear that go into an escape."

—CARL ANDREWS
INTERNATIONAL AWARD-WINNING MAGICIAN

Modern Day
HOUDINI

Secrets of My Twenty-five
Greatest Escapes

Bill Shirk, *as told to* **Dick Wolfsie**

THE LYONS PRESS
GUILFORD, CONNECTICUT

AN IMPRINT OF THE GLOBE PEQUOT PRESS

Cover and interior photos © Bill Shirk.
Text design: Casey Shain

Library of Congress Cataloging-in-Publication Data
Shirk, Bill.
   Modern day Houdini : secrets of my twenty-five greatest escapes / Bill Shirk and Dick Wolfsie.— 1st ed.
      p. cm.
   ISBN 1-59228-196-6
   1. Shirk, Bill. 2. Escape artists—United States—Biography. 3 Magicians—United States—Biography. I. Wolfsie, Dick. II. Title.

GV1545.S54S55 2003
793.8'092—dc22
[B]   2003054634

Manufactured in the United States of America
First Edition/First Printing

To my mother and father, Betty and Bob Poorman, who together made it possible for me to perform the ultimate escape, birth. My parents always told me to live my dreams and they have always supported me while I did just that.

I love you Mom and Dad.

Contents

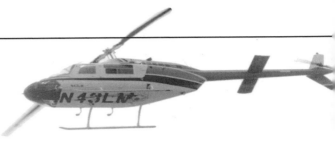

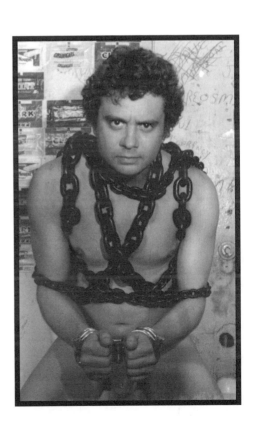

Acknowledgments

Thanks to all the wonderful people who took the photographs that have helped chronicle my quest to be the Number One Escape Artist in the World, especially Bill Moss, Gary Yohler, Tony Valainis, Robert Schaefer, Steve Kennedy, and the Milbourne Christopher Collection.

MODERN DAY HOUDINI

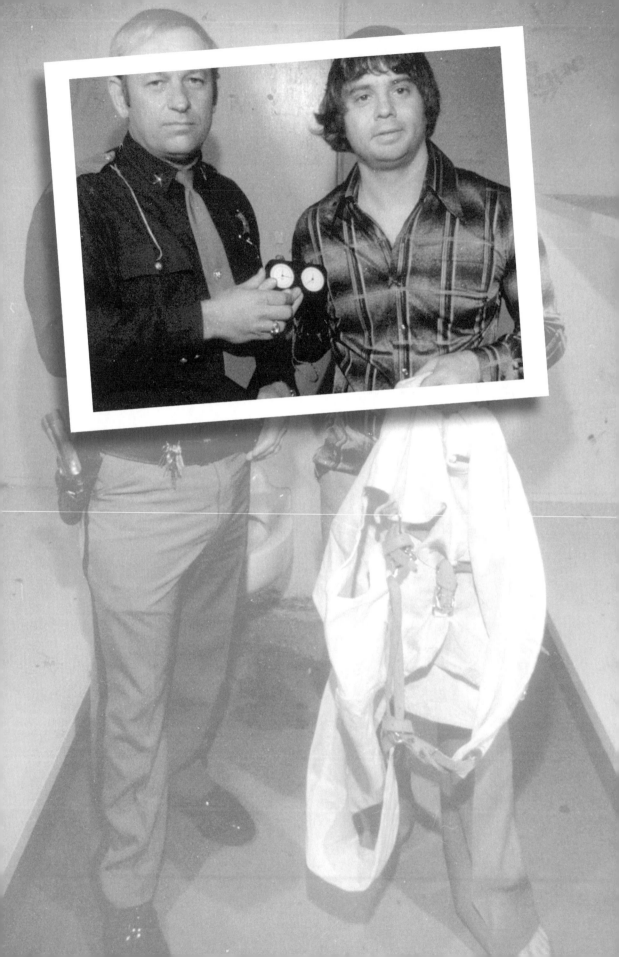

Introduction

MY NAME IS BILL SHIRK.

I am the number one escape artist in the world. I have held eight world records in escapology. For many years I also had the biggest ego in the world. The *Guinness Book of World Records* doesn't have a category for that. But trust me.

Some of that ego has worn off. Not all of it, though, or I wouldn't be writing my autobiography.

Ever since I was a kid and was locked in my basement with rats and a 14-foot python, I wanted to be an escape artist.

That isn't true, of course, but I'm desperate for an explanation for my life's work. I really can't find one.

I did always want to be number one at something. Anything. But why this?

I do know that from the moment I laid my eyes on Milbourne Christopher's book *Houdini, the Untold Story*, I was hooked . . . bagged, strangled, and buried.

Houdini paid his dues, and he ultimately became the highest-paid performer of his time. I tried to shape my escape career to mimic his. I think I have given it a pretty good shot. There are things I've done that the master himself never accomplished. Or even attempted.

And like Houdini, I made a lot of money. Not at first, but ultimately my sense of business and drama paid off. Of course, a lot of that money went to the IRS. There are some things you just can't escape.

As you read this book, you will question why any sane person would do the things I have done. I don't have a clue.

Yes, I wanted to build a radio and TV empire and to be fabulously wealthy. Others have had similar goals. But would they hang in a straitjacket by one ankle from a cable attached underneath a helicopter 1,610 feet in the air, be buried alive for two weeks with six rats, or have their head tied in a bag with a deadly rattlesnake? That's how bad I wanted it.

People have called me crazy my entire life. Read the book to see just how crazy I am. Let me know what you think.

> I do know that from the moment I laid my eyes on Milbourne Christopher's book *Houdini, the Untold Story*, I was hooked . . . bagged, strangled, and buried.

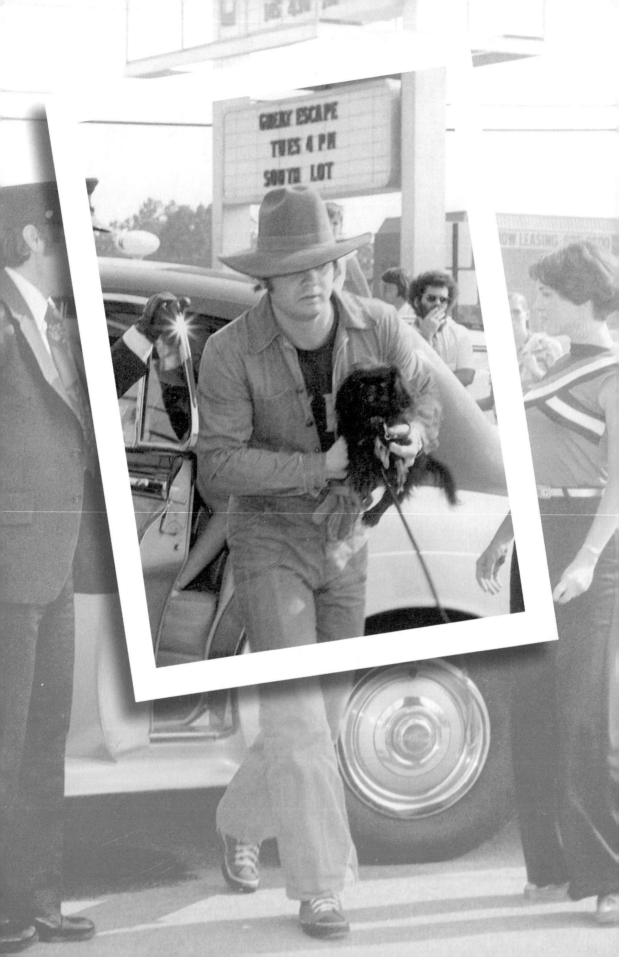

GREAT ESCAPE
TUES 4 PM
SOUTH LOT

NOW LEASING

Craning My Neck

IT WAS JUST LIKE ANY NORMAL DAY at radio station WXLW where I was the afternoon disc jockey. *Normal* might be the wrong word. Radio stations pretty much stay away from normal, always searching for the edge that will make them different. The television show *WKRP in Cincinnati* wasn't too far from reality, except for the Loni Anderson part. (What a shame.)

I had seen some crazy promotions during my ten years in radio. But on June 10, 1976, my life changed. And it all started with just another wild promotional idea—an idea that would turn my life around, upside down, and tie it in knots. Literally.

The request from event promoter Frank Powell seemed pretty straightforward—at least it did to him. He wanted me to do a fund-raiser for Variety Club charities at the Hoxie Circus, which was scheduled to be in Indianapolis in the next few weeks.

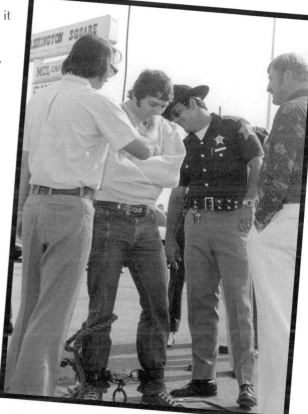

"I want you to publicize on your radio show that you're going to get in a straitjacket and allow yourself to be hoisted up off the ground 50 feet by a crane while your ankles are tied. Then you'll escape."

"What do you mean?" I said. Which was a pretty dumb response because it was crystal clear what he meant.

"Bill, get with the promotion. You're going to be like Houdini."

"You mean a stuntman, an escape artist? That is so cool. Can you teach me to do that?"

"I can't teach you that. No one can." He hammered this into me as though he sensed I was intrigued with actually doing it. "Bill, you're going to chicken out. There's a drummer in the band who does this kind of

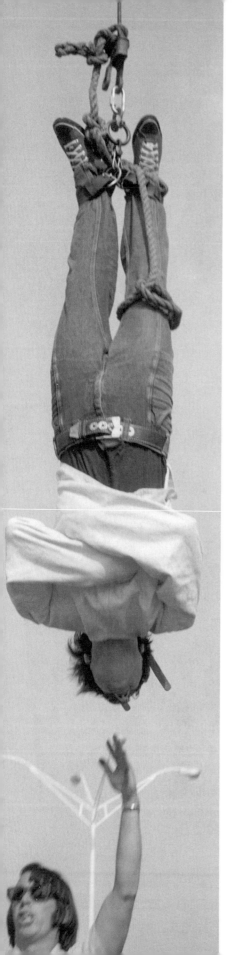

stuff. At the last minute you'll offer a hundred bucks for someone to do it for you. Then he'll step in. It's foolproof."

He stared at me when he said the word *fool*.

And so there it was. I was going to be the best example of a promotional chicken since Frank Perdue started advertising on TV. Okay, why not?

The next day I showed up on Old Joe Pickett's radio show. They'd even called him "old" twenty-five years prior. Radio is theater of the mind, so it was necessary for Joe to react when he saw what I was wearing . . .

"What happened to you?" he blurted out when he saw my arm in a sling.

I explained on the air that I had injured myself while practicing a daredevil stunt. Then I told Joe about my plan to get out of a straitjacket while hanging from a crane 50 feet in the air.

"No one is going to hoist you 50 feet in the air. Heck, I'll give you a hundred bucks if you pull this off," said Pickett.

The studio phone rang. It was Frank Powell. He'd been listening to the show, aware that I was going to be making an appearance. I should have known.

"Tell you what, Shirk," he said. "You get your butt down to the circus that day and I'll make sure you have a crane. The least I can do is give a friend a lift." Powell snickered and hung up.

Pickett tried to hide his smirk.

You can smell a good promotion a mile away. Powell was onto something. We both were.

The next day on my radio show, the bit hit the fans. Calls streamed in. "Go for it, Bill," many said. "Don't do it, Shirk, you're nuts," said others. "You'll get killed if you do that." It was hard not to have an opinion.

That's what good radio is all about.

Then it hit me. Hit me like a ton of wet cement— something I'd be hit with in a future escape. This entire promotion was based on a lie. It was based on my *not* doing what I'd said I would do. Suddenly I hated the whole thing.

I met with Powell that day. "I want to do the stunt myself," I told him.

"You want to do what? You can't do this. Are you nuts or

just crazy? Don't answer that."

The more I tried to convince him, the more ruffled he got. "Do you want to kill yourself? Don't answer that, either." He was turning a lovely shade of red.

Frank then asked a number of other questions he didn't want the answers to. The conversation ended with no commitment on my part either way. But I knew what had to be done. I needed to find a straitjacket and start practicing my escape.

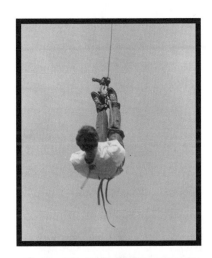

There were no magic shops in Indy in 1976. Oh, a few costume shops had packaged tricks, but I needed the real thing. *Chicago must have magic shops*, I thought. Sure enough, I found one in the Yellow Pages.

I called and told the clerk I was looking for a straitjacket. You could see his grin over the phone.

"Funny you should ask for that. I have a guy who wants to sell all his escape stuff—jackets, leg irons, cuffs, ropes, even books. Everything. And all for a hundred bucks."

"Why so cheap?" I asked.

"Well, he tried a straitjacket escape in a swimming pool and almost drowned."

"You mean you can get hurt doing this stuff?"

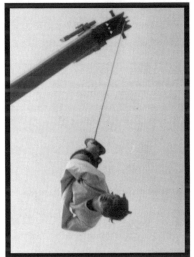

I was glad Frank Powell wasn't listening to this conversation. He would have asked: *Are you suicidal or do you just have a death wish?*

Two days later I flew to Chicago. I met the seller, a wiry little dude who gave me a brief overview of straitjacket escapology, then asked for my assistance in getting himself into the restraint.

The show began. And indeed it was a show. He began contorting his body, twisting, turning, grunting. Minutes later he had escaped.

"I could have done it quicker," he explained, "but that would make it look too easy. This is a show. Not a race. Learn from the master."

He meant Harry Houdini.

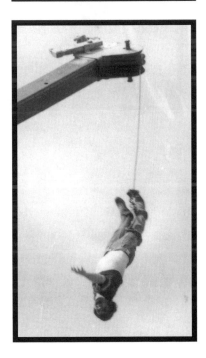

He put me in the jacket. Based on only one demo from the owner, I extricated myself in twenty-five seconds. Little did I know that this was only one second short of the world record. My wiry friend was astounded . . . flabbergasted at my speed.

But he cautioned me again to remember that it was all about show business.

Still, I was thinking: *Anyone can milk this sucker, but you don't read about guys who ran the five-minute mile.* I knew then that I could beat the world record someday. Even then some thoughts of being the Number One Escape Artist in the World started creeping into my egotistical head.

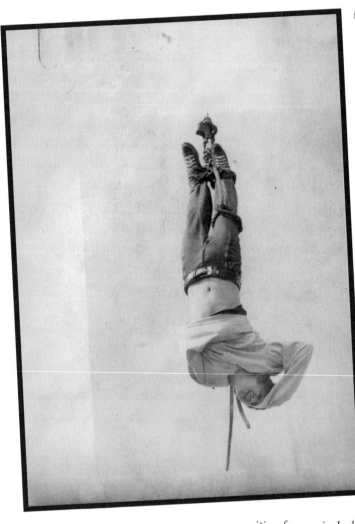

I still needed to learn that I had a lot to learn.

That evening I went to a local pub for a beer. While playing with a set of thumb cuffs I had purchased from the magic shop, I realized I was drawing a lot of attention. People just loved this stuff. And I loved being at the center of it all.

The next day I went to the local library. The name *Houdini* had started to obsess me, and I scanned the shelves looking for books about him or by him. *Houdini, the Untold Story* by Milbourne Christopher caught my eye. I didn't leave the library until I had read every word. I was hooked. But I had a long way to go. There was a crane waiting for me in Indianapolis.

The crane turned out to be my first problem. I knew I could get out of the straitjacket. In fact, I figured it would be easier upside down, with gravity helping. My problem was getting off the ground. The crane operator had been instructed by Powell *not* to lift me more than a few feet.

I gave the operator fifty bucks. That solved that problem. Now only the two of us knew what was going down—or going up, in this case. The rush of being in control was indescribable. Everyone's eyes were on me. When I asked for something, I got it. I was the center of everyone's universe.

It was a hot day. Very hot. I was placed in the straitjacket and the crane began to lift me. This was the first time I had ever been lifted upside down by my heels. The blood rushed to my head, the restraints tightened on my back as I was taken higher and higher. The pain in my ankles was excruciating.

Frank Powell was still in disbelief. He'd been so sure this was a foolproof plan. He had never met this fool.

I was right about the straitjacket. It did come off quite easily, but I remembered how important the show was. I milked the act for about two minutes. I could feel every eye on me. Especially Powell's.

"You're the craziest mother I ever met," said Powell when I was lowered to the ground. But in his heart, he knew this was the greatest promotion he had ever been part of. I knew it, too.

"You're the craziest mother I ever met," said Powell when I was lowered to the ground.

When asked by the media about my accomplishment, I was ready. "Are you listening?" I boasted. "I'm going to be the Number One Escape Artist in the World."

I meant that, every which way and Sunday. This was no bull, I told everyone.

And speaking of bulls, I take you to Escape Number Two.

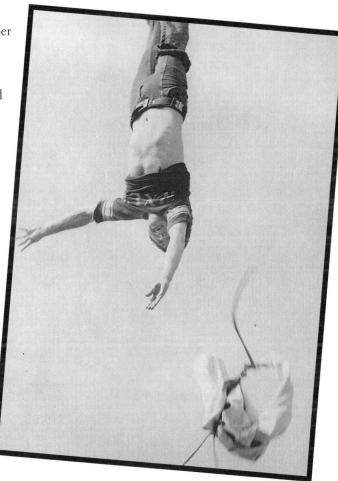

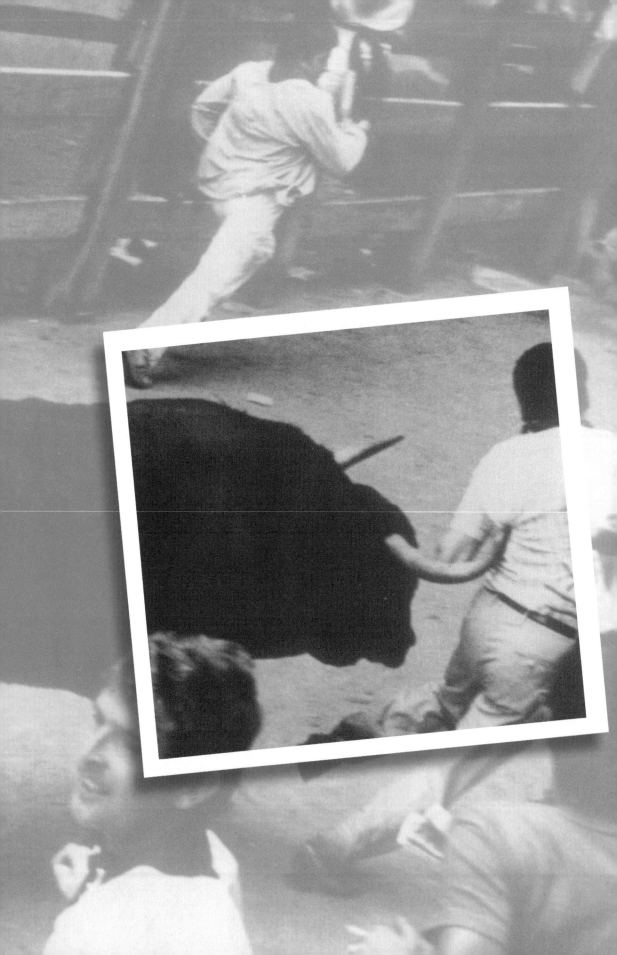

Horns of a Dilemma

THAT FIRST ESCAPE WAS A TOTAL EGO TRIP.
A recognition that I was onto something. Something big. What a blast to walk into a situation and control everything, everybody! To have people come and watch me perform. To hang on everything I said or did. Even when what I was doing was hanging.

Being an escape artist is all about ego. You have to have a huge one if you want to survive, but if your ego gets too big—if it gets bigger than your ability—you're a dead man.

I learned the hard way.

I knew after the first escape that hanging by a rope, upside down, from a crane, in a straitjacket at a local mall was not my entry into the Escapologist Hall of Fame. Not that there was such a place, but there was the *Guinness Book of World Records*, filled with numbers that proved, yes proved, that someone was number *one*. Yeah, I could call myself the greatest escape artist, but people could argue that. I didn't want any arguments. I wanted to be number one. If people asked me how I knew that, I could say: *If you don't believe me, look it up.*

The next step was to find a stunt—a word I hate, but who are we kidding?—a stunt that would set me apart, that would make me unique.

As a crazy twenty-one-year-old college kid, I had gone to Pamplona, Spain, and run in the streets with the bulls. This is ten days during the year when all those who love Spain, or those who wish to die by being punctured, scamper through the streets of Pamplona while a small herd of two-ton bulls horn their way down the narrow corridors looking for someone to skewer. Now at the age of thirty-one, I was older and smarter. Still crazy, probably, but this time I had a mission.

I convinced my brother, Bob, that this was the next step in my quest to be the World's Number One Escape Artist. My plan was to put on a straitjacket, run in the streets with the bulls, and, while doing so, get out of the restraint. Bob was not sure this was a good idea, but he was sure I was a taco short of a combination plate.

Bob and I both liked Spanish women. Time for a road trip. Pamplona, here we come.

Remember all that stuff about planning, about being in control, about total preparation before you do any escape? Do you remember all that?

I didn't.

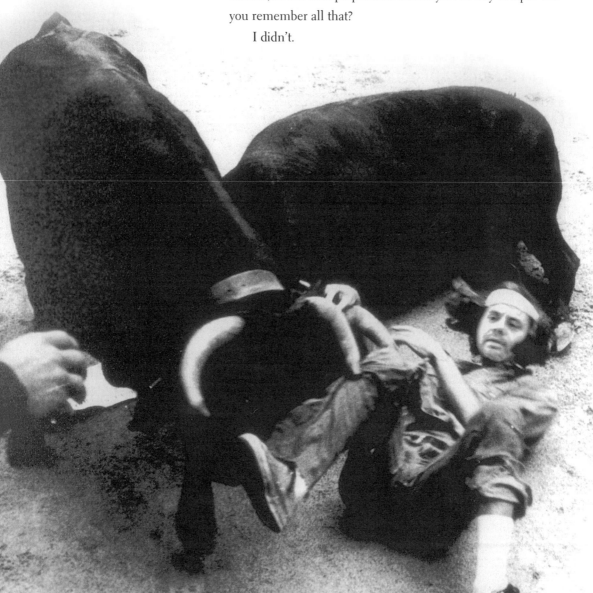

After landing in Madrid, I realized that we were still 1,250 miles from Pamplona, an eighteen-hour drive. I hadn't planned on that. We arrived in Pamplona. There were no hotels. I hadn't planned on that, either. It wouldn't be the first time I had slept in a car.

These seemed like only minor inconveniences, but they should have told me that I had not given this project enough thought. Truth is, I was in over my head. Way over. During the next few days, we scouted the place and got our bearings. Finally we were ready to enact our plan. Not that we had a plan.

The streets of Pamplona are packed with people prior to the running. This made it easier for my brother to put the jacket on me without drawing too much attention while I "lost" myself in the crowd. I wasn't sure at this point if the straitjacket would cause any commotion.

I didn't have to wait long.

The cannon sounded and hundreds of people dashed into the street, screaming at the top of their lungs in anticipation of the bulls sweeping past them. My brother had lodged himself in one of the corridors along the street where runners crowded to see the action but avoid the danger.

Bob's job was simple. Or so I thought. Just get a photo of his little brother barreling down the street, twisting and turning, while trying to get out of a straitjacket and avoid the equivalent of being run over by twelve SUVs with antlers.

I didn't want to be ungrateful, but it seemed to me I was the one doing the hard part.

I was running alongside a man with a huge gash in his forehead. He was using several safety pins to hold his face together. This was not a good sign.

Bob was good at shooting the camera, but lousy at holding it. The camera was knocked from his hand as the bulls herded past me and I stripped off the jacket.

He never got the shot of me.

The next day we tried again. This time I decided to pause near where Bob was standing as the bulls and people stampeded past me. Because I was in the straitjacket, I couldn't run very effectively. Truth is, I had more of a chance

I was running alongside a man with a huge gash in his forehead. He was using several safety pins to hold his face together. This was not a good sign.

of being trampled to death by the Spanish mob than being gored.

Bob situated himself on the other side of the fence barricade, even farther from the charging bulls. Now it appeared as though we had orchestrated it perfectly. This time, however, I decided to shed the jacket earlier so I could run more effectively. I scampered through the streets, avoiding each bull, extricating myself from the restraint.

I did witness one man horribly gored in the back by one of the bulls. My inclination was to think this guy was crazy. Can you imagine what he would have thought about me?

But I was home free. Or so I thought.

Reveling in my own success, I turned toward my brother for some positive feedback. Apparently, however, two of the bulls had slipped on their own droppings when let out of the gate (this is probably more information than you wanted). Suddenly those two bulls, slightly behind schedule but wanting to make up for lost time, headed toward me.

I was literally caught between the two animals, wedged between their horns and suspended several feet off the ground. *God, I hope we got this picture*, I'm thinking. *And I hope I'll be alive to see it.*

I fell to the ground and picked up the straitjacket.

Not a good idea. The Spaniards saw the jacket and thought it was a cape, a prop that is strictly forbidden during the running of the bulls in the streets. This is such a cultural gaffe that I was soon pummeled by the local populace, convinced I was responsible for the bulls' reckless and erratic behavior.

Even while I tried to escape, I was obsessed with the photo. No picture, no proof, no chance to be the World's Number One Escape Artist.

I looked for my brother. Again, he'd lost the camera in the excitement. He'd also lost a front tooth. The local police had seen enough. Bob and I got an escort out of town. And I learned something about the Spanish legal system: In order to avoid any jail time in Pamplona, you need either a very good lawyer or a $1,000 Pulsar watch. Enough said.

Now, how about that photo? I wasn't going back without

I was literally caught between the two animals, wedged between their horns and suspended several feet off the ground. God, I hope we got this picture, I'm thinking. And I hope I'll be alive to see it.

one. Bob and I walked the streets of Pamplona, photo-less and bull-less, when there in a store window we spotted a local newspaper. And on the front page was a photo of me, an incredible shot taken by some guy who was obviously smart enough not to hire his brother as a photographer.

"How hard would it be to get a copy of that photo?" I asked the clerk.

"Very hard, señor," he said.

"How about if I gave you a hundred bucks?"

"That would make it much easier, señor." Luckily, he didn't need a watch.

I had my second escape fully documented, and I had a brother who thought I was fully demented. Only now, looking back (something that I should have done about ten seconds sooner that day in Spain), do I realize how close to death I was.

We took a vacation down in Costa del Sol. It was time to think about Escape Number Three.

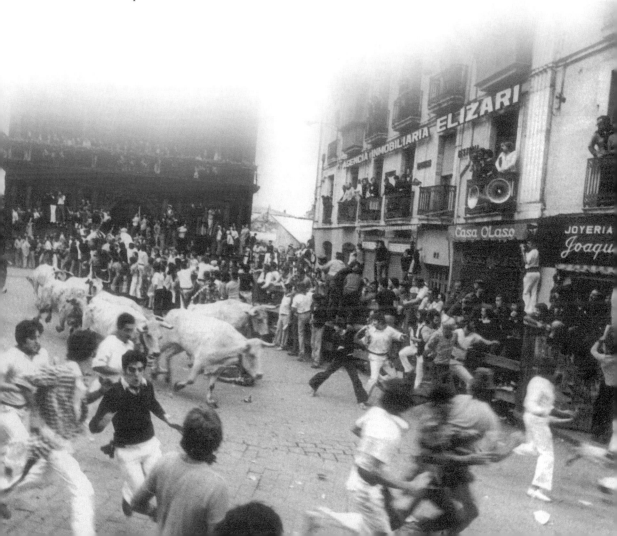

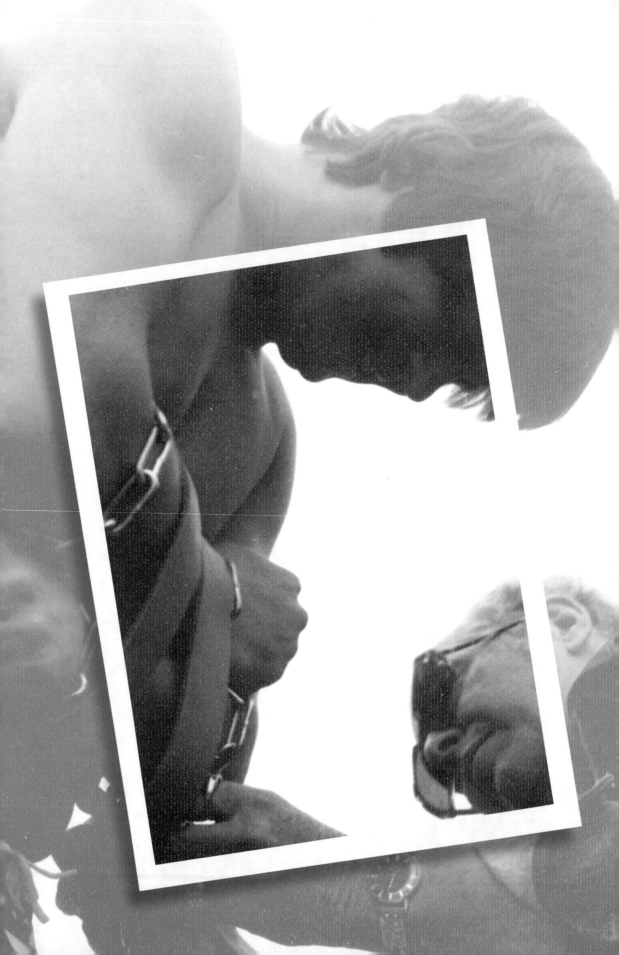

Bridge Over Troubled Water

IT WAS DIFFICULT TO ENJOY THE PLANE RIDE back from Spain. I was aching in more ways than one: Aching from the free lift I'd gotten from a couple of two-ton bulls and aching to find another escape that would make my dream of becoming the Number One Escape Artist in the World a reality.

Back home, some people, including my parents, were already questioning my sanity, and some wondered about the effect my daredevil behavior would have on the radio station's credibility. People thought I was nuts.

I'm not sure I minded that. That image had great public relations possibilities. It also sold a lot of radio time.

I knew one thing. With people walking on the moon and flying around in space, my escape from another straitjacket would not garner the attention I needed. I thought the photo of me in the streets of Pamplona dodging bulls would create more of a stir. Ultimately this escapade would become part of my

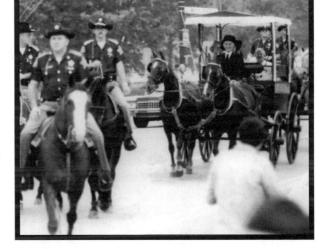

myth, but in the early stages it didn't play out the way I wanted.

Still obsessed with the life of Harry Houdini, I continued to read every book I could get my eyes on, searching for ideas for my next escapade. Houdini had hung from several buildings in his career. In 1925, he did it at the old Indianapolis News building in front of 26,000 people, but my efforts to secure permission for a feat like that were in vain.

I came up with a better idea. One of Houdini's most popular escapes was to jump from a bridge, often in some kind of shackle, an escape that newspapers covered and his fans flocked to see.

That's what I wanted: TV, radio, and newspaper coverage. And a couple of thousand people watching me risk my life.

I knew I could pull it off. I knew I could jump off. But—as you'll see—my planning was a little off.

I was convinced that a straitjacket was becoming a bit commonplace, and I had also learned that escaping from a straitjacket in the water was like opening a car door in a submerged vehicle. The pressure against the jacket makes it virtually impossible to extricate yourself. I needed a unique eye- and ear-catching restraint. And one I could get out of.

One of the contraptions I had purchased in Chicago several months earlier was called an Australian Torture Belt, a device used by the English during the colonization of Australia to restrain prisoners. I liked the sound of it. Again, great PR value.

Ironically, of course, the guy was selling the contraption because he had almost killed himself trying to get out of it underwater. A bargain to die for. I also discovered that I was pretty good at getting out of the device, despite the convoluted series of straps and restraints. At least on land I was pretty good at it.

Now I needed a bridge.

I was convinced that a straitjacket was becoming a bit commonplace, and I had also learned that escaping from a strait-jacket in the water was like opening a car door in a submerged vehicle.

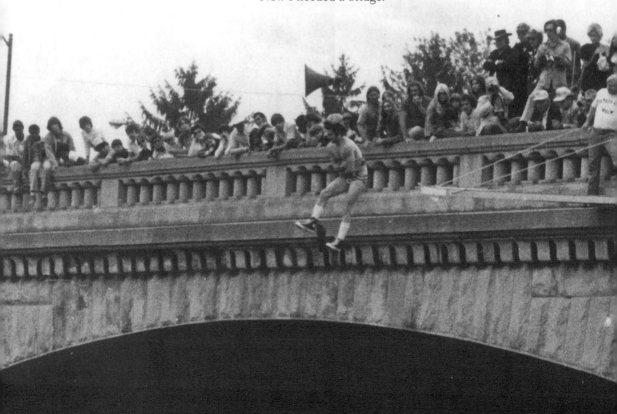

I chose the 30th Street Bridge in Indianapolis, a gothic structure with a stone facade that harked back to the days of Houdini. It was perfect. (Actually, it was far from perfect, as you'll see.)

At that point I figured I had thought of everything. But here's a list of the top ten things I hadn't thought of:

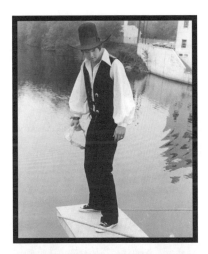

10. Getting permission to do the jump.
 9. Health and liability insurance (with a rider for water damage).
 8. Knowing how cold the water was.
 7. Knowing where the rocks were.
 6. Knowing whether I could get out of the belt underwater.
 5. Being sure I would sink when I hit the water.
 4. Knowing whether I would survive when I hit the water.
 3. Having a plan if I was drowning.
 2. Knowing how long I could hold my breath after a jump.

And the number one thing I forgot:

 1. Knowing how deep the river was.

David Letterman, eat your heart out.

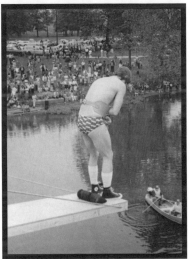

When I told Frank Powell my plan, he asked if I was crazy. I was used to this by now, but he did scare me into thinking about some of the safety issues. Frank also helped secure permission from the city for me to take my life in my hands. In today's world I'm not sure a city would grant permission, but within two weeks I had the document in hand.

Frank also convinced me that my harebrained idea of wearing a brimmed hat with a balloon inside filled with air was ridiculous. This was my solution for how to breathe underwater.

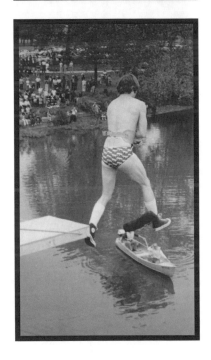

"Sure, you can try that, Shirk," he said. "But remember, you'll have to tie the hat on your head with a strap under your chin. Then, when you hit the water, the force of the water under the brim will propel the hat upward and your head will come off."

Frank has a way with words. I dumped that idea.

It was time to practice the escape. And it was time to get my brother back in the picture. Not that he was very good with pictures. But Bob did know something about water and was a certified scuba diver—whose brother, Bill, was gaining quite the reputation as certifiable himself.

Bob and I scoped out the bridge. It was 35 feet above the water's surface, but the jump from that bridge would land me in about 3 feet of water and onto a number of huge rocks—an immediate roadblock to my initial idea of staying underwater for a couple of minutes while I escaped. If the river dropped any more, it would have been my first mud escape. Either that or the jump would kill me.

Bob and I worked to clear the river of rocks, but it soon became apparent that the channel was several feet in front of where I would land. I needed a way to jump farther out into the river.

My engineers at the station constructed a platform so rickety that just standing on it made me question the entire idea. I realized that I was going to walk the plank. Literally. Nice image.

It was time for my first practice jump. At Bob's suggestion I had tied an anchor around my ankle to be sure that when hitting the surface I would sink into the river, whereupon I would escape from the Australian Torture Belt unseen by the crowd. If there was a crowd.

I stood at the precipice (of both the bridge and my career). I had put on the belt to get a sense of the fall with additional weight. My heart was racing; I was having second thoughts, then third and fourth thoughts. My brother jolted me back to reality. "I thought you wanted to be the Number One Escape Artist in the World," he reminded me.

Enough said. I jumped.

I hit the water at a comfortable angle. It was easier than I had thought. *Success!* An hour and four beers later, I tried the jump again against my brother's advice. Was the bridge wobbly? Or was it me?

This time it seemed like I crashed the surface with even more force, but several feet off the mark and into only about 4 feet of water. The agony was intense. I had severely sprained my left ankle.

The doctor said that if I stayed on crutches and didn't do

My heart was racing; I was having second thoughts, then third and fourth thoughts. My brother jolted me back to reality. "I thought you wanted to be the Number One Escape Artist in the World," he reminded me.

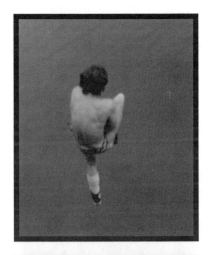

Five Things Harry Houdini Taught Me

1. The secret of showmanship is not what you do but what the mystery-loving public *thinks* you do.

2. Don't be upset that some people come to see you fail or get hurt. Or die.

3. Always have a second way out or backup plan in case you screw up.

4. Physical fitness and a healthy diet are musts. Stay in the right mental and physical condition to succeed. [Note from Dick Wolfsie: Shirk is full of it. He ate a cheeseburger after every escape.]

5. Boldly go out in front of the crowd and tell them what you are going to do. (Perhaps the audience will believe you.)

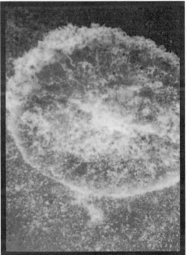

anything foolish for several weeks I would be okay. And if I didn't stay on the crutches, then I would be on crutches for the rest of my life. Huh? Oh, the hell with the crutches.

For two weeks prior to the jump, I would use the crutch as a crutch, pumping the publicity and piquing the public's interest. I just hoped that on the day of the event, no one said, "Break a leg."

The day of the escape arrived: September 25, 1976. It was a gloomy day. Almost depressing. Houdini would have been proud of me. I was dressed in a pseudo-cowboy outfit and carrying a shark's jaw; I arrived in a stagecoach with several pretty girls alongside me. On second thought, maybe he wouldn't have been proud of me.

He would have been proud of one thing. I had drawn an enormous crowd, including fourteen mounted policemen. All the publicity from TV, radio, and the newspaper had quickly rekindled people's memories of my earlier feats. There were close to 3,000 people there. I arrived thirty minutes late, building the tension in the crowd. I know Houdini would have liked that.

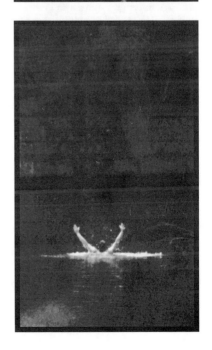

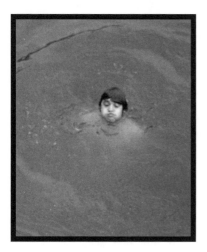

The third time I came up to a thunderous ovation. I was free of the belt, free of the anchor, and free to pursue my next escape.

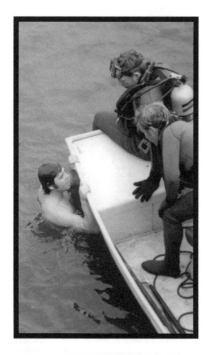

I sensed the beginning of true recognition as an escape artist. Yes, I could draw a crowd. But could I do the escape? I had probably spent too much time planning the wrong end of this entire thing.

I carefully made my way over the bridge railing and out onto the platform. I screamed to the crowd, asking if they wanted me to be successful. A huge roar went up. Then I asked how many didn't want me to make it. The roar was even bigger. Fine with me. Whatever works.

As I stripped to a bathing suit, a local locksmith wrapped the leather and chains around me and put the padlocks in place. A sheriff's deputy tied the anchor onto my left foot, which was still swollen like a tennis ball.

Here was the plan: I would jump into the river, sink to the bottom with the help of the anchor, squirm out of the Australian Torture Belt, and surface within two minutes. I had never planned on unlocking the padlocks. That wasn't necessary, but I knew people would assume that's what I'd done. So be it.

Read that last paragraph again. Most of that never happened.

I looked down. Frank Powell had arranged for a complete safety crew, including an ambulance and a scuba diving team. This was supposed to make me feel more comfortable. Maybe he didn't think I could do this.

I picked up the anchor and limped to the edge of the rickety platform. My ankle throbbed with pain. I feared the anchor would twist me into some unspeakable position and I would injure my back when I landed.

I jumped. *Smack!* I hit the water flat on my back, my rear end taking most of the impact. The wind was knocked out of me.

Worse, the anchor (a bag of sand) came off my ankle. I found myself floating to the surface, the worst thing that could happen from the standpoint of an exciting escape.

I desperately began to paddle my good right foot, hoping to resubmerge into the murky water. But it was necessary to exhale what little air I had left, otherwise I wouldn't stay under—the air in my lungs would bring me to the top.

Under the icy water I realized how little time I had, but managed to free myself of the belt. It sank to the bottom of the riverbed.

I went up a second time for air, reenacting the myth of the man who comes up three times before he drowns. My nose got a big round of applause. But this was no act. My body buoyancy was driving me to the surface. Getting some air was a nice bonus. I had made a number of mistakes planning this event, but this deserved an Oscar for acting and improvising.

The third time I came up to a thunderous ovation. I was free of the belt, free of the anchor, and free to pursue my next escape.

If you'd asked me then, I'd have said the stunt seemed to last an eternity, but if pushed I would have guessed that it took four minutes. It was the next day in the paper that I learned for the first time that my entire escape had taken forty-seven seconds.

The longest forty-seven seconds of my entire life.

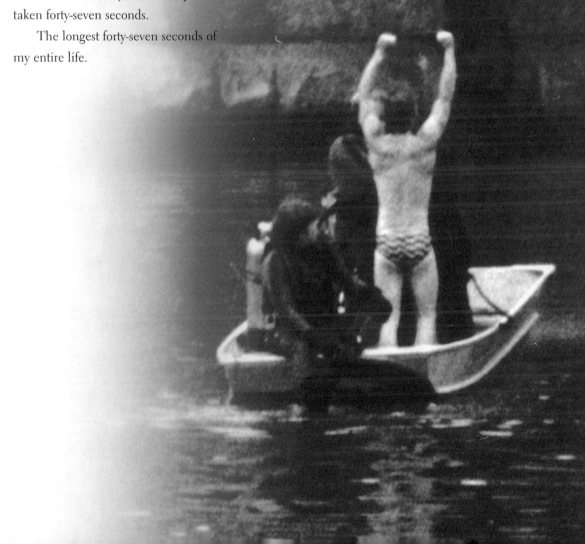

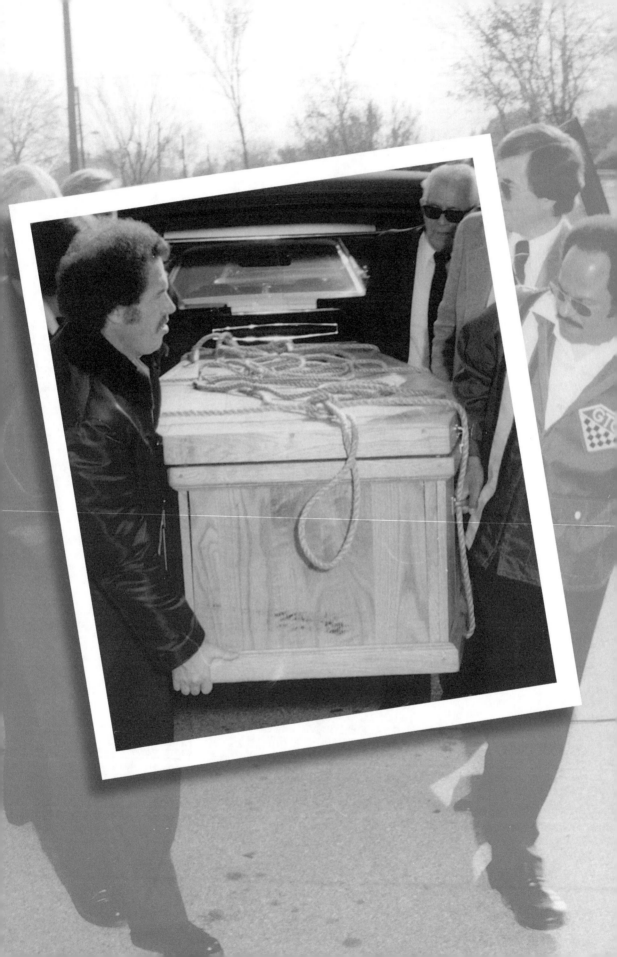

Life in the Underground

I WAS TAKING ONE ESCAPE AT A TIME. But I knew that each escape needed a "hook." There had to be some method to the obvious madness I was displaying.

Fall in Indianapolis—where the signs of Halloween begin with pumpkins, scarecrows, and witches popping up in windows and on doorsteps in early October. I knew from my Houdini reading that the golden anniversary of the master's death was Halloween 1976, the perfect date for a caper.

But what to do? I needed something scary, eerie, almost macabre, and worthy of the world's greatest showman who had died fifty years earlier.

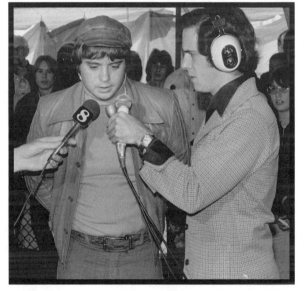

To establish myself the equal of Harry Houdini, I would need to surpass him in some areas. One daredevil act that Houdini had never warmed to was being buried alive. He had tried it once near the Pyramids in Egypt, but he was almost killed and found the entire process a bit much psychologically, even for him. Said Houdini: "The next time I'm buried, I'll be dead."

If I could achieve something that Houdini had not been 100 percent successful with, I would be on my way to becoming the Number One Escape Artist in the World.

Yes, I would bury myself alive.

Truth is, I never anticipated actually being underground for very long. I saw the whole thing as an illusion. That's what magic is all about. I wasn't going to be buried alive. I would have a tunnel that led me to a motor home. I'd talk to the press on phones from the RV. I wouldn't spend ten minutes buried alive. Did they think I was crazy?

Oh, yeah. They did.

Frank Powell of Variety Club Tent 10, again promoting the event, was adamant that he would not be part of something

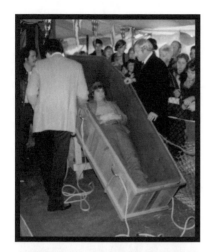

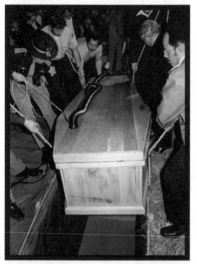

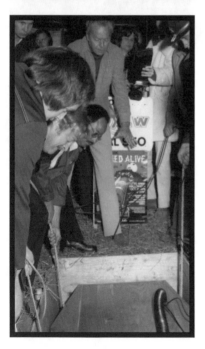

that was essentially a fraud. "If Variety Club's name is on this, it's got to be real."

Looking back, this was the best advice I ever took. True, escape is an illusion, but if this deception had been divulged, the pure nature of the trickery would have meant the loss of public trust and a real drag on my growing fan base. A false accomplishment does not get you into the *Guinness Book* or make you the Number One Escape Artist in the World.

Yes, this was the correct decision, but at that moment I was experiencing a full-blown case of claustrophobic paranoia—almost as if trapped right then and there. I had explored caves and dived in underground caverns, but as Houdini found out, the whole concept of being interred creates a psychic dread. I was feeling it.

This didn't stop me from beginning an aggressive promotional campaign on the radio. The very sound of "Bill Shirk Buried Alive" created a huge response. Phones rang off the hook. Radio listeners wanted more information; the media wanted interviews; spiritualists wanted me to talk to Houdini while I was down there. It was all unreal. But it was supposed to be.

Next I needed a hole in the ground, bigger even than the hole I was digging for myself on the radio show by claiming I would do this. I couldn't back down, but knew I would soon be let down, very slowly, into my grave.

I chose some land that I owned near 30th and Kessler in front of WXLW and solicited the help of two station engineers, Horace Smith and Jut Reuter, who despite being near retirement age thought this whole thing was a hoot and wanted to be part of the action. Horace and Jut dug the grave site with pick and shovel. No backhoe, all muscle. It took a week.

Now I needed a coffin. Sensitive guy that I am, I started calling mortuaries and funeral homes. And I did it on the radio during my live radio show. That's me, Mr. Politically Correct.

Funeral directors, not widely known for their sharp sense of humor, did not find this funny. No one was going to sell me a coffin for a stunt like this. Truth is, in those days, if you weren't dead they wouldn't even talk to you about a casket.

One way of judging a friend is whether he would build you a casket. That is a friend who will be true to the end. Literally. Mike Perry was a friend. He built me a coffin in three weeks. Oak slats, gothic looking. It was a beauty. Drop dead gorgeous.

We decided that rather than just lower the coffin into the hole and cover it with dirt, we needed a rough box so that in an emergency the dirt above the coffin could be extracted from the ground quickly.

This rough box was actually another larger box that the coffin fit into, thus making it easier to secure the air source and communications lines. Above the coffin when it was placed in the rough box were a wire screen and a tarp connected to the cables and straps on top of the grave. In theory this meant the dirt could be lifted out quickly in an emergency rather than requiring that it all be removed by hand. This was the theory, anyway. I didn't spend much time testing our theories. I learned the dangerous way.

There were three phones: one to the surface of the grave, which was connected to a public address system; one for emergency purposes; and one for me to talk to the media around the world. Despite what some media were saying, I did not have a death wish. I wanted to be buried alive and unburied alive.

Folks on top could talk to me on a Mickey Mouse phone, the first one produced by Disney. That's how we got money for charity. Talk to Shirk in his grave on the Mickey Mouse phone and make a contribution.

Walt Disney would have rolled over in his grave— something I would be able to do in about two days.

To get air into the coffin, we used a vacuum cleaner with an exhaust hose slipped through a hole in the coffin lid. When the vacuum ran in reverse, it sent fresh air into the casket. Well, kinda. Stay tuned.

No food, and no water. That simplified things and made for better press. I had cleaned out my system and taken a few pills to clog up my plumbing. I know, I know, too much information.

Two days before Halloween. I arrived at the grave site in a hearse. Out of the hearse came six pallbearers carrying a coffin. The coffin opened, and inside was a gorgeous young lady. The crowd loved it. (Let me tell you, talking a girl into a coffin is harder than talking a girl into bed.)

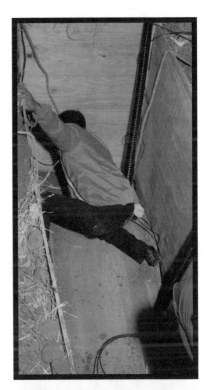

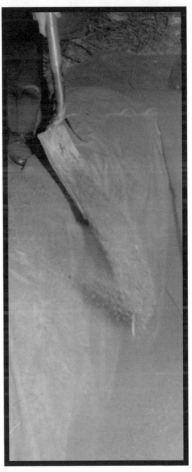

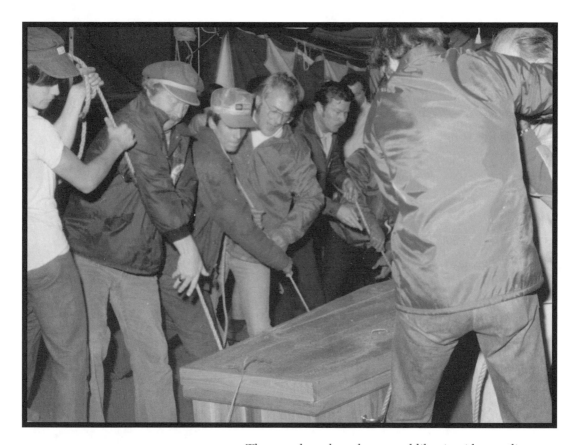

My public responded,
but this time, unlike the
bridge jump—when
they were looking for a
mishap—they must
have related to my
predicament. "Dig him
out," they screamed.
"Dig him out."

The crowd was hyped, pumped like ringside wrestling fans, ready to rumble. I was going to wrestle with death. And I hoped I was the favorite. I got into the casket, a very, very strange feeling.

As the coffin was lowered into the ground, I began feigning agitation and claustrophobia, pretending I was on the verge of completely freaking out. As dirt covered the coffin, I began screaming: "Dig me out, dig me out." It boomed out over the public address system above.

My public responded, but this time, unlike the bridge jump—when they were looking for a mishap—they must have related to my predicament. "Dig him out," they screamed. "Dig him out."

Frank Powell never misses a cue. He walked over to the microphone and pretended to calm me down. "It's okay, Bill. Everything is going to be okay. We're all up here for you. You can do this. It's all for charity, Bill."

What an actor.

Now I'm underground. No room to move. I'm on my back. My finger in front of my nose. Total darkness. Very humid. I'm

sweating. I try to organize my tiny space, moving the phone
wires, trying to get comfortable. It's getting more humid.

I ask the crew to pump in fresh air. But the compressor, the
reverse vacuum, is sitting on the freshly dug ground, and its
initial gust of cool air fills the coffin with dirt and grime.

Now I'm hot, dirty, and in total darkness. The beginning of
a very long forty-eight hours.

In my tiny space I could hear almost everything from
above. Like an Indian scout putting his ear to the ground, I
found that the noise above was almost a thundering whisper,
vibrating down to me.

Time had already ceased to exist. I had not brought along
a watch, thinking that my obsession with the passing of each
minute would make things worse.

A Shirk in a box. In a box! You won't believe what
happened next.

I fell asleep. But no nightmares. Being awake was the
nightmare. Suddenly tremendous
pressure on my chest. Was it a heart
attack? No, worse!

**One of the wooden
crossbeams that
supported the coffin lid
had split from the
weight of the dirt and
was pointing toward my
heart like a dagger. I
screamed, convinced
I would be crushed or
skewered to death.**

One of the wooden crossbeams
that supported the coffin lid had split
from the weight of the dirt and was
pointing toward my heart like a dagger.
I screamed, convinced I would be
crushed or skewered to death. Above
me, the volunteers confirmed that the
dirt had caved in about a foot above the
grave. They weren't sure what to do.

Finally volunteers hitched two
cars to each side of the tarp and wire
mesh connectors and pulled it tight,
relieving the pressure on the coffin lid.
I quickly broke off the crossbar and put
it aside.

The media was all over me like
dirt on Shirk. I spoke to radio stations
around the country: Los Angeles, New
York, Chicago. I was on the phone
twenty hours a day.

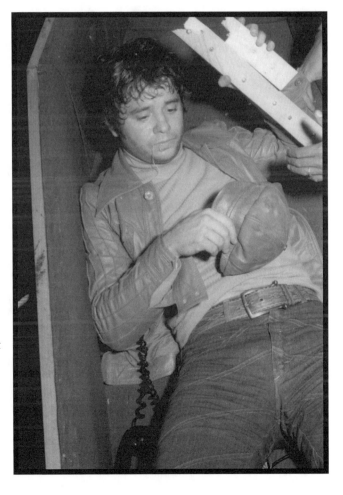

Newspapers from everywhere. Australia, Japan. Even the *New York Times* wanted to do an interview. I was in heaven—although I was actually closer to the other place.

The electrical storm the second night had a devastating effect on everything. It started a small fire at ground level that sent smoke down into the coffin through the vacuum cleaner. The compressor had to be turned off, cutting off my air supply. At that point I figured I had about an hour left.

Then another nightmare. I heard the crowd above screaming, "The tent is collapsing, the tent is collapsing." I was trapped. Helpless. At that point there was no quick way to rescue me. I was scared. Very scared.

Eventually the tent was reestablished, and the fire was extinguished, but not my fears. I wondered what would happen next.

I had calculated my exit from the coffin to coincide with the time of Harry Houdini's death. Digging began at 1:30 P.M. Half an hour later, after the dirt was removed, the tarp and wire mesh were pulled off the top of the coffin. Through the slats in the lid of the coffin I could see daylight for the first time in forty-eight hours.

Then the lid came off the coffin. *It was like an atomic blast.*

I was hot, dirty, hungry, and thirsty. I felt worse than I had in the bar in Pamplona. I staggered out of the coffin. There were no muscles left in my body.

The crowd went wild.

I was held up by Frank Powell and Paul Scheuring, a newsman from WXLW. Paul had announced my departure from the grave to a huge listening audience as well as 1,000 people on site for the exhumation.

I inhaled a McDonald's cheeseburger, fries, and a shake.

There was $5,000 in the donation jar, money we had collected on site when people talked to me in the grave.

It was over.

No it wasn't. It was time to think of a new escape.

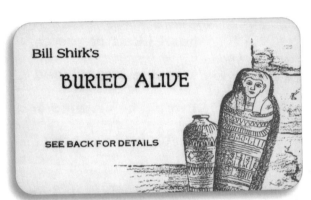

Bill Shirk's

BURIED ALIVE

SEE BACK FOR DETAILS

I had calculated my exit from the coffin to coincide with the time of Harry Houdini's death. Digging began at 1:30 P.M.

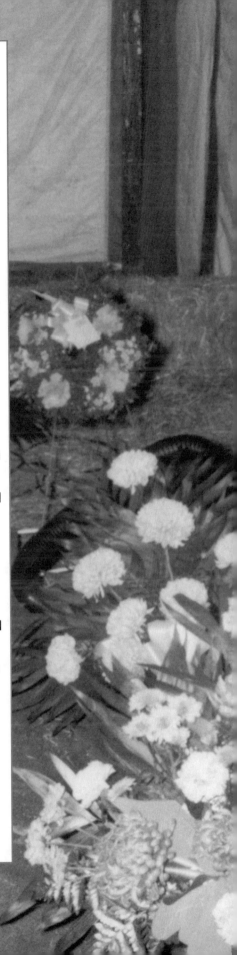

Five More Escapes Commemorating the Death of Harry Houdini

1. (Halloween, 1979) I was entombed in a block of cement with two rattlesnakes, two tarantulas, and no food or water, remaining there for eighty hours. The public viewed me through a glass window in the block of cement. Raised thousands of dollars for charity. Two thousand people at Lafayette Square witnessed my breakout with the help of a jackhammer.

2. (Halloween, 1980) Marvin Johnson, undisputed world boxing light-heavyweight champion, tied me up in 100 feet of rope at the Indiana State Fairgrounds. I then hung 20 feet in the air, upside down, from my ankles. Twelve minutes later, despite severe pain in my ankles and serious rope burns, I freed myself from the ropes.

3. (Halloween, 1995) At Fountain Square in Indianapolis, I was handcuffed and chained and then hung 20 feet in the air from triple burning ropes. Within two and a half minutes, I escaped from the restraints after two of the ropes had burned in two. Had the third rope burned in half, I would have fallen and likely broken my neck.

4. (Halloween, 1996) I sat in a chair and allowed people to tie me in 100 feet of rope. I've done this on numerous occasions; it was one of Houdini's favorites. When they finished tying me in the chair, I kicked off my shoes and used my feet to gain slack in the rope. I tipped the chair back and forth, eventually falling over and escaping. Once I tipped too far, fell off the stage, and was knocked unconscious.

5. (Halloween, 1999) This was my upside-down straitjacket escape record, breaking Mario Manzini's record of 8.5 seconds on the national TV show *Guinness Games.* To commemorate the seventy-second anniversary of the death of Harry Houdini, I escaped from a straitjacket in 3.47 seconds while hanging upside down, but I never officially registered my performance.

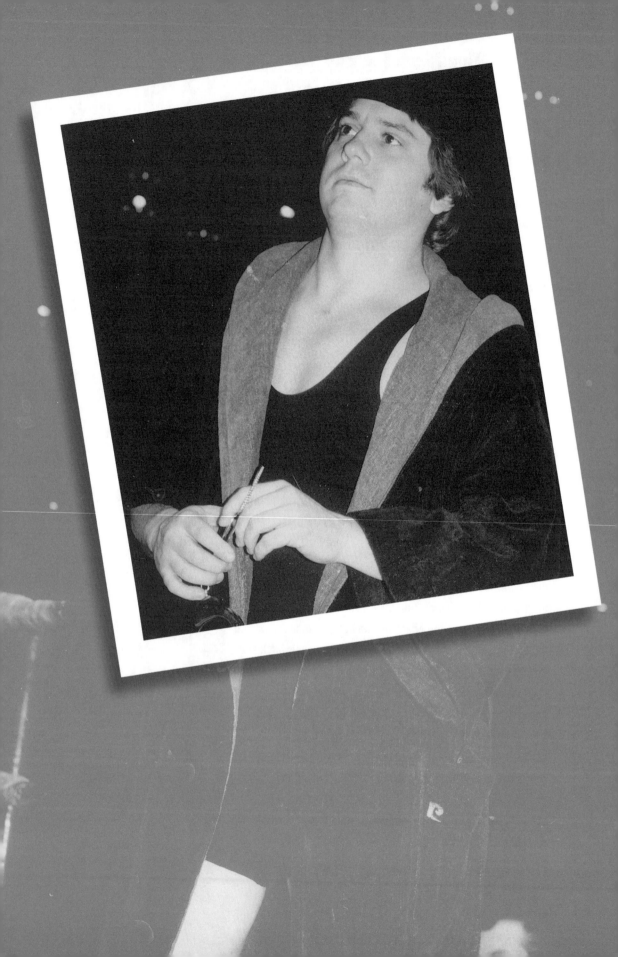

A Fighting Chance

IN ESCAPOLOGY THERE IS A BLURRING between what is
real and what is illusion.

Think about a magic trick. You know it's a trick. A coin
can't really disappear. But you respect the artistry that created
the illusion. After a magic trick most people ask themselves (or
the magician) how it was done, but absent the answer, they are
content to just enjoy the skill they have just witnessed.

It is the same with my
escapology. People wonder how I
did it. A few may question if I
really did it, but ultimately they
just love seeing it.

Which brings me to
professional wrestling. And why
I was a big fan.

Wrestling is similar to
escape artistry. The illusion of
reality is the basis of a successful performance. Most
wrestling fans know that it's
only entertainment, but they
would no more question it
than they would a movie or

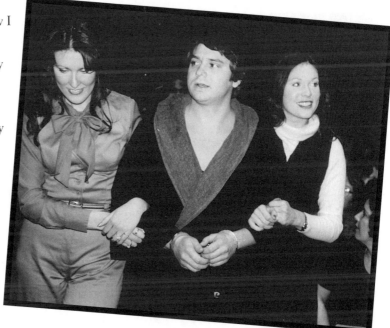

theatrical performance. You can cry at a movie. Why can't
you boo a wrestler?

Spectators can enjoy the performance on a number of
levels. In the case of wrestling and escaping, the unforeseen
and the unplanned are aspects that keep the crowd on edge.

So why am I talking about wrestling?

In many ways it seemed a good way to further promote
myself and still use a few escape techniques. Plus I desperately
needed some video of my work.

Back at WXLW Joe Pickett had, at my urging, unleashed a
brilliant promotional idea with nationally known wrestling star

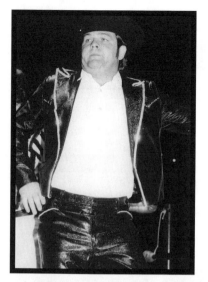

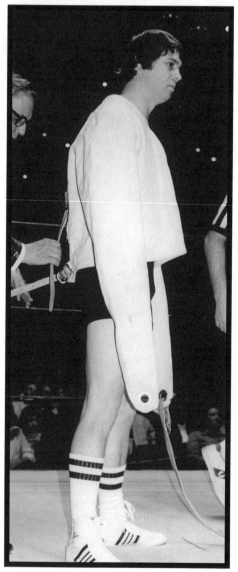

Dick the Bruiser. Pickett had set up a mock wrestling match on the radio between himself and Bruiser. Once again, here was illusion at its finest. Were they really wrestling on the air? Was that really an ambulance the listeners heard in the distance? No difference. You could enjoy it no matter what you believed.

The promotion worked so well that fifty people were lined up at the radio station to see the match, which we had promoted as taking place in the basement of our building. We didn't have a basement.

Yes, the wrestling phenomenon was sweeping the country and was alive and well in the Midwest. In fact, Bruiser lived right here in Indianapolis. Was there a way to capitalize on Bruiser's celebrity?

I called Sam Menacker, general manager of All Star Wrestling, and ultimately set up a meeting with him and Dick the Bruiser. At the meeting I begged Bruiser to let me be involved in some kind of professional wrestling promotion.

Now, Bruiser was used to people begging him. People begged him not to break their arms or crush their legs. People in his own neighborhood begged Bruiser not to turn over their cars with his bare hands. In general, Bruiser did not warm up to begging.

Plus Bruiser suffered from a heart condition. He didn't have one. At least not in the ring.

But incredibly, Dick agreed to set up a match between me and a wrestler named Cashbox, a spiteful, vicious, and dangerous man (those were middle names) who had actually heckled me at the bridge jump in Indy. What I didn't know was that Bruiser had arranged that. Bruiser had already hitched his star to me, recognizing that the drama of my escapes had promotional value for wrestling.

Bruiser may have looked mean and dumb. But he was just mean.

Here was the concept: I would be restrained in a straitjacket, and Cashbox would have one wrist handcuffed to the ring pole. A $200 check would be placed in the center of the ring, and the first guy to reach the check would own it. I agreed to give mine to Variety Club Tent 10. But I don't think Cashbox, despite his name, was out there to raise money for charity. He had already bragged that he was going to beat me to a pulp. First, though, he was going to kick out my teeth.

Bruiser made it clear how dangerous this would be and that Cashbox was not going to pull any punches, an expression that had obviously lost its metaphorical humor with me.

In order to set up the promotion, Bruiser introduced me to the Saturday-night wrestling fans just before a scheduled title tag-team bout. During the festivities Cashbox and his assassins, the Bounty Hunters (the world tag-team champions), jumped into the ring and tried to rough me up. It couldn't have been any rougher.

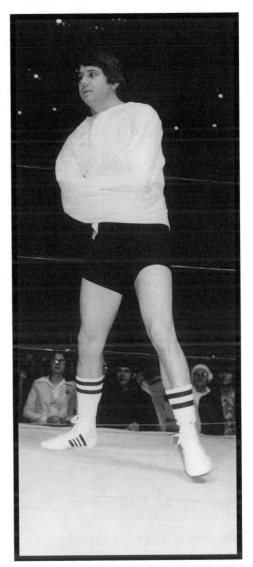

After three endless minutes wrestlers Spike Huber and Bruiser jumped into the ring and saved me. They wanted me to stay alive so I could die the next time. I admired their promotional sense.

The big night arrived at the Indiana Convention and Exposition Center. For all the talk about wrestling being fake, prearranged, and planned, it was kinda scary to me that I had been told NOTHING. I had no idea what was supposed to happen. I realized that a herd of half-crazed bulls was more predictable than a full-crazed wrestler who clearly didn't like me.

Before the match the referee asked me for a key to the handcuffs I had provided "so in an emergency, Cashbox could get out." I knew better. I was being set up so Cashbox could pulverize me.

I gave the ref the wrong key. On purpose. This was about as scared as I had ever been. I was taking no chances.

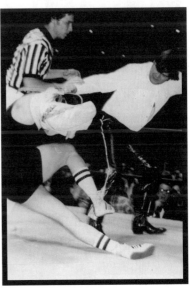

A police officer secured me in my straitjacket, and Cashbox's one wrist was handcuffed. The other cuff was supposed to go around the ring post, as I said, but it didn't fit and so was simply attached to the top rope.

Bad idea! I should have been a little suspicious. Maybe I was just paranoid.

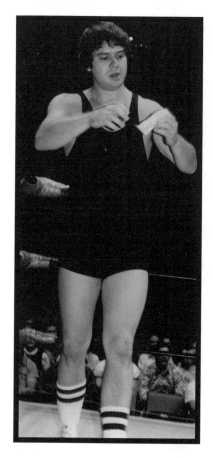

The ring announcer introduced us. Cashbox generated heat, meaning that people hated him. Of course, that's what he wanted. Six thousand people rose to their feet and booed. I got a huge round of applause. Why? Because I was nuts enough to do this, that's why.

The bell rang. In the grand Houdini style, I began rolling around on the floor trying to build tension before the escape, pretty convinced I could stretch this out a bit. And remember, I had the right key. Cashbox would not get out of the cuffs.

But Cashbox didn't have to get out of the cuffs. He simply moved down the ring while the cuff was still secured on the top rope. He was like a rottweiler on a dog lead. With no muzzle. He actually had access to almost half the ring, despite being tethered by one wrist. My suspicions were correct: Just because you're paranoid doesn't mean people aren't trying to pulverize you.

Cashbox kicked me in the back several times. Next he grabbed my hair. Then he got bored and crushed my nose. Remember, I was still in a straitjacket. For him, it was like beating up a mummy.

Finally I got out of the jacket, retrieved the check, and began taunting Cashbox, who by now had gotten the false key from the ref. He wasn't happy. He was still handcuffed. I got my butt back to the dressing room. The crowd was on their feet cheering me.

I was thinking that I should leave town for a decade. That would have been my smartest escape so far.

But apparently, Cashbox recognized the promotional value of what we had done—or Bruiser told him to recognize the promotional value of what we had done—and he agreed to another match. This time we would both be in straitjackets, but Cashbox's restraint would have only one buckle fastened in the back, while mine had the normal four.

Here was another bad idea. Your grandmother could get out of a straitjacket with one buckle. Well, *my* grandmother could. I taught her well.

Six weeks later we wrestled again. Cashbox wasted no time. He was out of the jacket in seconds, then wrapped it around my neck to choke me. All the time he was pummeling my stomach

Cashbox kicked me in the back several times. Next he grabbed my hair. Then he got bored and crushed my nose. Remember, I was still in a straitjacket. For him, it was like beating up a mummy.

with his fist. You ask: Were these fake punches? Honestly, Cashbox would probably have said yes, or I'd have been seriously dead, but tell that to my 175-pound body. It hurt!

What else could go wrong? Lots! Spike Huber leaped into the ring to help me. In the tussle I accidentally smacked Cashbox in the head with my straitjacket. The buckles chipped Cashbox's tooth and split open his lip. This was not part of the plan.

Not that I remember having a plan.

Incredibly, this stunned Cashbox and he fell. I jumped on top and pinned him. If there had been a plan, this would not have been part of it.

Again, I was thinking a trip to Spain might be a good idea. I was petrified that Cashbox was going to clean my clock. He wasn't happy. In the dressing room he was bleeding and in a rage. But Dick the Bruiser stepped into the potential fray. "Don't be a pussy," he carefully explained to Cashbox, as he gently slammed him against the wall. "Mistakes happen."

Bruiser had a way with nerds.

I would perform a few more times for All Star Wrestling, but it was time to move on.

Actually, I was lucky I could move at all.

What else could go wrong? Lots! Spike Huber leaped into the ring to help me. In the tussle I accidentally smacked Cashbox in the head with my straitjacket. The buckles chipped Cashbox's tooth and split open his lip.

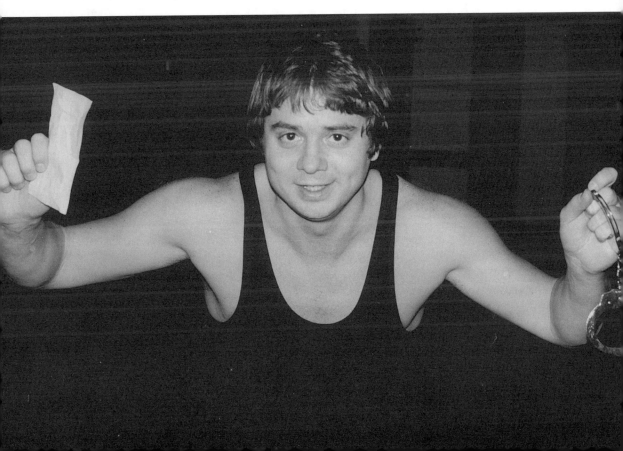

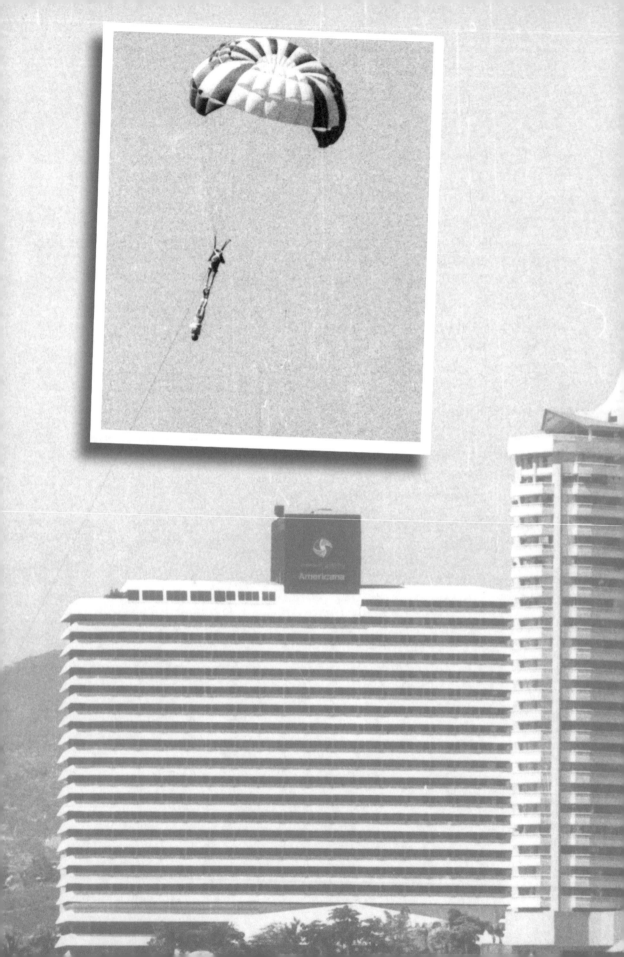

That Jumpy Feeling

MY NEXT ESCAPE WAS MOTIVATED by a show
I saw on ABC. *Wide World of Sports* was featuring the natives
of Mexico diving off the cliffs of La Quebrada in Acapulco.
That's all I had to see.

Show me something breathtaking, then give
me a straitjacket, and I'll really take your breath
away.

Escape artists and kids have one major thing
in common: It's almost impossible to get
permission to do something dangerous. Over the
years I've been more tangled in red tape than I
have in pythons and arm restraints.

Would someone let me jump off their cliff?
Wait a second. Can someone even own a cliff? I
didn't want any trouble from the Mexican
government. I figured a Mexican jail was pretty
much like a Spanish jail, but the water was worse.

Bob and I arrived in Acapulco, only to learn
that amateur cliff jumpers were not welcome.
Kids and escape artists also share an unmistakable
stubbornness, so we continued our search for the
perfect cliff.

Just a few miles north were more cliffs,
higher cliffs, more dangerous cliffs, more
isolated cliffs. More reason to want to do it.

Bob and I walked to the edge of one
precipice and peered over. The view was so
picturesque that the dangers it held eluded us for
the moment. An eerie sparkle seemed to
emanate from the cliff walls. Unfortunately, the
glow wasn't so much majestic as it was Corona.
The effect was caused by thousands of beer
bottles that had been cast away by locals and tourists who were
enjoying both the view and a brew or two. I knew the broken
glass was a potential problem.

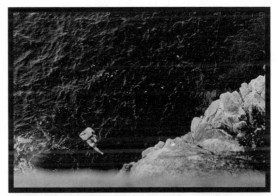
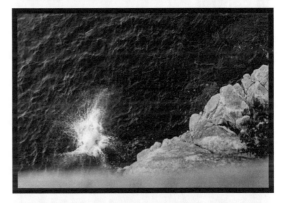
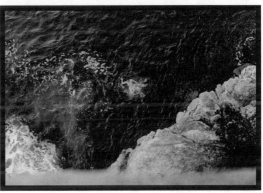

> **And how about that straitjacket? The idea here was to get out of one, not die in one. The jacket restricted my momentum during the jump and further compromised my ability to control my flight.**

Remembering the bridge jump back in Indy, Bob and I took some careful measurements to ensure that I would clear the cliff walls when I jumped. This would require a pretty hefty hurdle on my part, maybe as much as 15 feet straight out from the ledge to guarantee hitting the water.

Even tougher to gauge was the water's depth, which changed based on the tide and the movement of the waves. I made some careful calculations that assured me I would land in a sufficient amount of water. That's if I jumped at the right time. Big *if*.

And how about that straitjacket? The idea here was to get out of one, not die in one. The jacket restricted my momentum during the jump and further compromised my ability to control my flight. If I were injured, it would be quite a while before anyone would be able to reach me.

The morning of the jump I felt at ease, possibly a false sense of security fostered by the beauty of my surroundings. In all fairness, Bob and I had spent a substantial amount of time calculating the jump. We had left no stone unturned, except for the millions that waited for me beneath the surface.

Remember, however, that there is no point in practicing a jump like this. Once you do it, you've done it, which sounds like something Yogi Berra would say.

I walked to the edge of the cliff. I looked over. The view

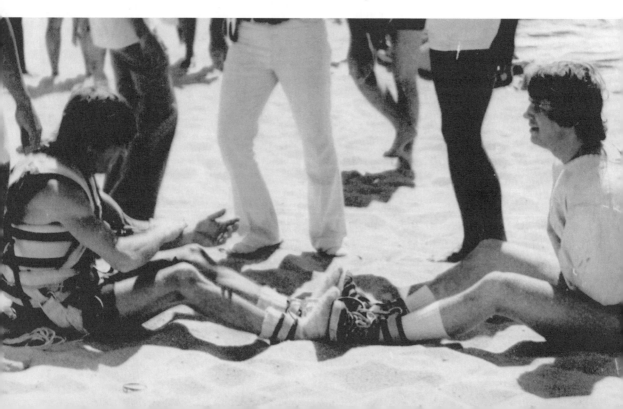

made the jump off the bridge in Indianapolis seem like a step into a bathtub. Except my bathtub didn't have a ton of broken glass in front of it. I carefully cleared the area, giving myself a path to begin a running jump.

Bob secured me in the straitjacket. Remember, this was the straitjacket I had purchased in Chicago from a guy who'd almost killed himself in his own swimming pool when the jacket became wet and waterlogged.

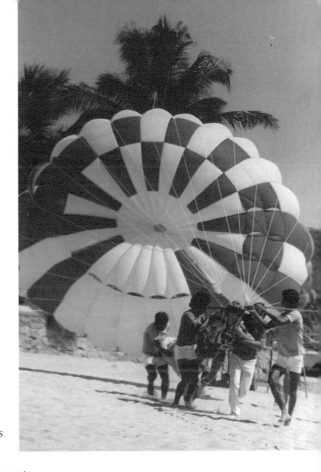

That was in his own pool. I was 150 feet up and 2,000 miles away from my own swimming pool.

I jumped!

I fell through the air at what seemed a blinding speed, but with 150 feet to drop, the time seemed almost endless. On impact, the wind was knocked out of me and I quickly sank. The straitjacket quickly absorbed the water. It was no longer just a restraint. It was an anchor. I longed for chains and locks, which now seemed easy to negotiate compared to a soaking-wet straitjacket.

But I didn't panic.

I knew that to escape the jacket I would need to use a great deal of oxygen. The restraint was not only wet, but salty, too, creating an adhesive effect. I had freed one arm when a huge undertow actually assisted me in freeing myself of the jacket by pushing it away from my body. In the meantime I had been scraped along the bottom of the ocean bed. Glass, stones, and debris ripped into my skin. So many things were happening at once, I wasn't sure what to be the most scared about.

I kicked off the ocean floor, forcing my body to the top. Relieved as I was to suck some sweet air, I remember praying that Bob had taken the photo. That's what this was all about.

I was bleeding, I was exhausted, but I was elated. I made my way back up the cliff using shoes that I had previously lowered to the bottom of the bluff.

More than any previous escape, I felt good about not only its execution, but the preparation as well. As with all escapes, I was just glad it was over.

I fell through the air at what seemed a blinding speed, but with 150 feet to drop, the time seemed almost endless. On impact, the wind was knocked out of me and I quickly sank.

Of course, I still wasn't satisfied. Hey, I was in Mexico. *Let's not waste a minute*, I thought. It was time to head for the beach.

On the surface, parasailing doesn't seem very dangerous. Of course, you're not on the surface when you parasail. You're 50 to 500 feet above the boat, hanging from a kite, attached by a rope. The boat is usually driven by a guy understandably more concerned with what is in front of him than what's above him. Sometimes it's a beer that's in front of him.

Nevertheless, the idea of dangling from a parasail while escaping from a straitjacket seemed an appropriate, almost poetic way to end my Mexican holiday. I imagined myself gently swaying in the Mexican sky, dancing with clouds and conversing with the birds. In a straitjacket, of course.

It sounds corny, but it sounded good to me.

Finding someone to take you parasailing is easy. If you don't find him at a resort, he'll find you.

I found Jose, a local businessman just as adept at salsa as

On the surface, parasailing doesn't seem very dangerous. Of course, you're not on the surface when you parasail.

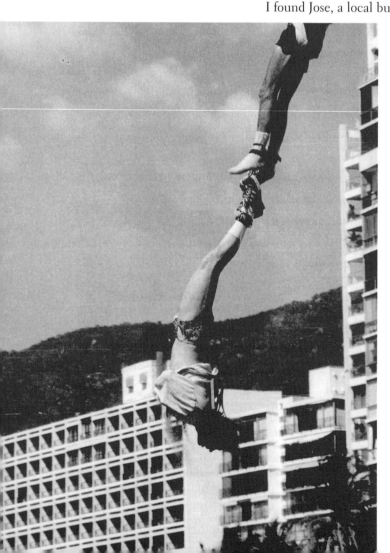

sailing since his local restaurant also took tourists on assorted boating adventures. I told Jose of my plan, and to convince him of my competence I showed him press clippings from my previous escapes.

"Are you loco?" he asked. Obviously a relative of Frank Powell's.

In fact, Jose remained skeptical of the whole idea until he learned of my burial escape, a feat that totally freaked him out and convinced him that I had magical powers. Then I offered him fifty bucks. That was apparently about as much magic as he could stand. We had a deal.

I knew then I had to call on my brother, Bob, for support. Literally.

Working with Jose, we decided that the best way to make this happen was for Bob to be strapped into the parasail, just like any tourist. With one *huge* exception: I would then be tethered to Bob's ankles, upside down, in the straitjacket. We would be staring at each other as the boat rocketed along Acapulco Bay, 500 feet in the air.

It seemed like a no-brainer, so I was the perfect person for the escape.

The next day we were ready to try it. It was ninety-five degrees, and humid. I was sweating like a Mexican pig. My straitjacket had dried out from the cliff jump, leaving a residue of salt. When the jacket was placed on my bare chest, it felt like I had been painted with Krazy Glue—a real problem if my goal was to extricate myself in record time.

We had enlisted the help of a few airline people who were staying over in Acapulco. One of the pilots even agreed to film the entire escape with his 8mm camera. "I hope you have one of those little black boxes on you," he said in a Mexican accent. Very funny.

Jose jumped into his boat and gunned it. The sail lifted quickly. But I didn't. Instead, I was dragged along the ground for about 50 feet, the terrain filling my swimming trunks with beachfront. It was also filling my mouth, eyes, ears, and nose with sand, glass, and pebbles.

As we gained altitude, the sand sprayed from my trunks, blasting Bob and me in the face. Even worse, the weight of my body was straining Bob's ankles and the straps were cutting into his crotch. Bob bellowed for me to begin the escape quickly, but ironically, any additional movements I made just increased the pain in Bob's ankles. And his face. And his crotch. This escape had seemed like a no-brainer. Now I was afraid it was going to end up a no-brother.

I desperately tried to free myself, but the jacket, so sticky from salt and sweat, was like another layer of skin and resisted my contortions. The harder I tried, the more painful it was for Bob. He was screaming. Of course, he was just my brother, but escape artists have feelings, too.

There was another problem. I had no communications with the driver of the boat. His cue to head for land was when

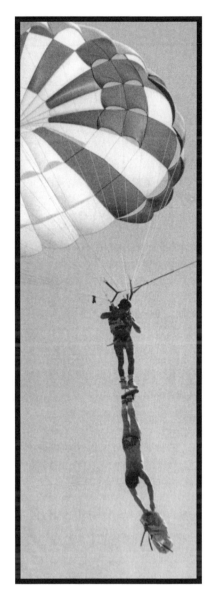

This escape had seemed like a no-brainer. Now I was afraid it was going to end up a no-brother.

I got out of the jacket. What if I didn't get out of the jacket? Then I would have a new world record: longest time spent in a straitjacket 500 feet in the air without getting out. Not what I was looking for.

Ironically, the stiffness of the jacket ended up being a plus. Once I freed one arm, the tautness allowed me to slide out of the remainder of the restraint rather than having to peel the jacket off. Total time to get out was just under fifteen minutes, a very, very long time for a pure straitjacket escape, but I had to do it while virtually glued inside and staring into the face of my brother, whose manhood I was sacrificing for this escape.

On paper this escape may not seem scary or dangerous, but some have died parasailing when the rope holding the sail broke. The participant could drown when he hit the water and be smothered by the sail. The weight added by our jury-rigged contraption made this a real possibility. I tried not to think about it. I tried not to think about anything.

The approach was tricky. There was concern that I would land on my head as we came down, which would have provided me with an excuse for my next fifty escapes. I hoped Jose's people were more adept at landings than takeoffs. There was no room in my suit for any more sand and glass.

Then it was over. Crowds of people who had peppered the beach gave us a huge round of applause as we landed and hoisted Bob and me onto their shoulders. This was a good thing for Bob, who had effectively lost all his ability to walk. At that point I wasn't sure if he had lost any other abilities. And his ankles looked the size of my ego.

Bob promised he would never help me again, a promise I respected. But I talked him out of it two beers later.

For all its beauty and grace, this escape had been hard on both of us. Nevertheless, we had great photos and some breathtaking film. Plus Jose brought Bob and me back to his restaurant for a burrito as big as our heads.

Jose wouldn't take the fifty bucks for the ride, but each burrito cost $39.95.

Then it was back to the hotel for two days. Our bodies were battered, yet our egos were unbruised. One more success, but miles still to go before I could claim the title of the Number One Escape Artist in the World.

There was another problem. I had no communications with the driver of the boat. His cue to head for land was when I got out of the jacket. What if I didn't get out of the jacket? Then I would have a new world record: longest time spent in a straitjacket 500 feet in the air without getting out. Not what I was looking for.

My Brother, the Escape Artist

By Bob Poorman

Whenever I tell people who my brother is, they question his sanity. I find this kind of strange. Of course, Bill *is* nuts. Does a sane person go underground for three days with a boa constrictor around his neck?

Look up the phrase *a method to his madness,* and there's a photo of Bill next to it. The truth is, Bill always knows exactly what he is doing.

In fact, it was for that very reason that he picked me to help him with his escapes. Bill knew that whoever assisted him with stunts had to be someone he trusted completely. Not just somebody who was taking the photos, but someone who truly cared about his safety and well-being. And not someone who would benefit from his life insurance policy.

We were pretty typical brothers, sibling rivalry and all. He'd wrap a python around his neck, I'd wrap a bigger python around my neck. Just kidding.

I do think the years we worked on all the escapes brought us even closer together. Sometimes it was much too close—like when Bill was tethered to my ankles underneath a parasail in Mexico.

I'm a marine biologist and I've led a pretty adventuresome life myself. But I'm getting older now and am slowing down a little. Most of the things I've done with Bill fall under the category of "Once Is Enough."

And if you've been reading this book, you'll see that in some cases once was a little too often.

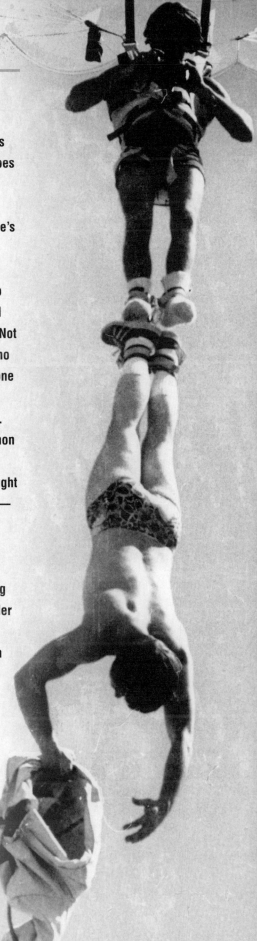

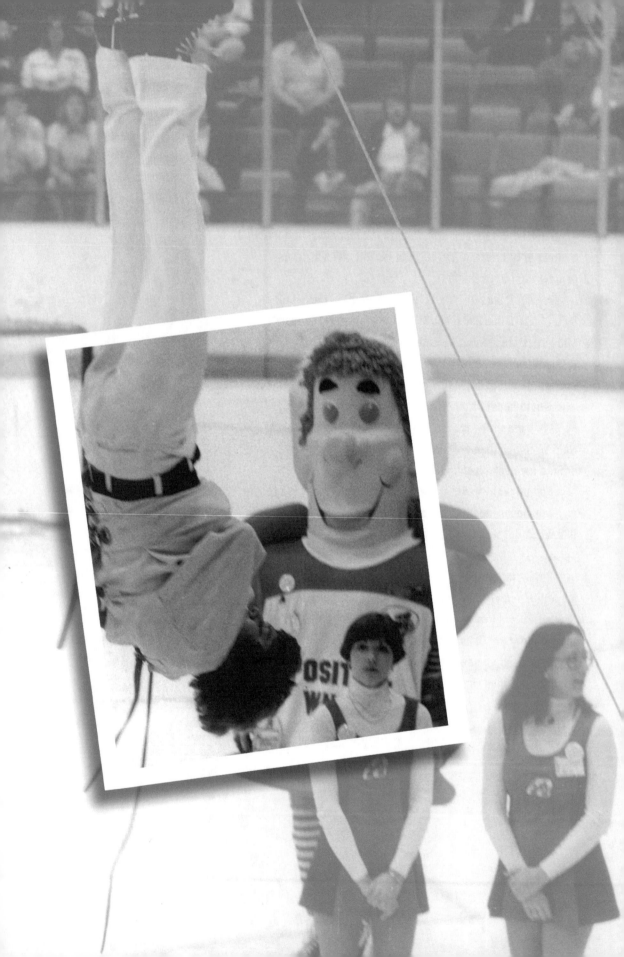

Facing the Crowd

AS I'VE SAID (TOO MANY TIMES), Harry Houdini was
the greatest performer of his time, maybe of any time. Even
without the mass media available today, Houdini was a
household name. His performances attracted thousands and
thousands of people. Most were eager to see
him succeed; others were not as generous.
But they came. Lots of them.

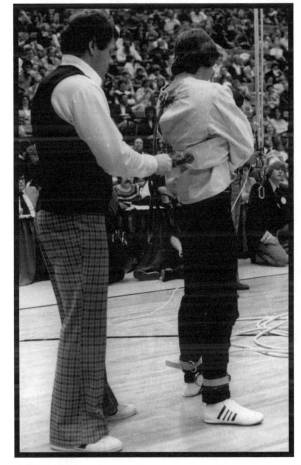

My frustration was that I had not
attracted huge numbers of people to my
events. I may have been a little hard on
myself, of course. Many of my escapes were
not devised for the public. You can't get a
crowd when you are on top of a cliff in
Mexico, or in a casket. Ten thousand people
were not going to camp out waiting for Bill
Shirk to rise from the earth.

In retrospect, it is also possible that I was
still lacking a bit in confidence. I knew if I
failed, it was better to do it in front of 300
people than 3,000 people. Or 30,000.

It was now the beginning of the 1978 pro
basketball season, and my friend Frank
Powell (yes, it's Frank, again) was now
involved in finding halftime entertainment
for the Indiana Pacers, the fledgling NBA
team that played at Market Square Arena.

As luck would have it (I get a fair share of that), the Pacers
game was to be televised on CBS—the first time that the
network would accord such a privilege to our team. Was I
drooling over this opportunity? What do you think?

The Pacers were playing the Bulls, a rivalry that had
already begun to blossom, and a sellout crowd was expected.

My plan was to perform the upside-down straitjacket
escape while hanging from a rope attached to a block-and-

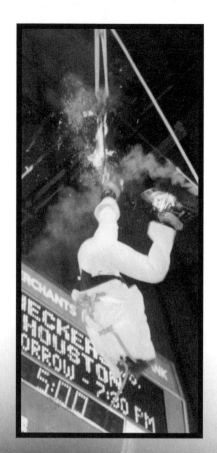

tackle secured to one of the catwalks that extended under the roof of the arena. As always, things looked a lot easier—and safer—on paper. But if I fell, I would hit the hardwood floor from 100 feet above the arena. There were Pacers who had hit the hardwood floor from 6 1/2 feet and were out for the season.

I realized the importance of dependable apparatus, so I enlisted the help of wrestler Spike Huber who—excuse the expression—knew the ropes when it came to this arena.

We settled on a simple configuration of ropes and pulleys—one that was safe, but would allow the twisting and turning necessary for me to free myself from the jacket while remaining suspended in the air. I had a vision of falling headfirst into the basket. *Swish.* Two points. (There were no three-pointers in those days.)

We practiced. I slipped into the ankle harness and attached it to the lower pulley. Spike gently lifted me into the air. I began to spin like a top—the opposite of the problem we had anticipated. Spike continued to pull on the rope and I continued to rise. And spin. Then, suddenly, I wasn't moving at all. I was flat-out stuck.

An escape artist stuck like that in front of 10,000 people is kinda like a tow truck plugged in the mud. Very embarrassing. It took twenty minutes for me to shimmy up the rope and back to the catwalk, with time to think about a better arrangement. Twisting and sticking were two things we needed to avoid.

We did avoid them. By using guide ropes extending vertically on either side of the lower pulley, I could prevent an inevitable spin every time I moved to free myself from the jacket.

The game was that night. I was proud of myself for carefully planning the escape. But you can't prepare for 17,000 eyes staring at you. I don't think the basketball

players feel that. There are lots of
players; the action moves around the
court quickly. But I felt that every gaze,
every stare, every skeptical sneer was
focused—like a laser—right on me.
And I was still on the ground.

Pacers star Billy Keller strapped me
in the straitjacket. It was a nice change
from my brother or a sheriff. Slowly I
rose, the spotlights hitting me in the
eyes. I could hear the hushed crowd.
(Okay, that's another thing Yogi would
say, but that's how it felt.)

I struggled for two and a half
minutes (two minutes of that was fake
struggling) and finally tore off the
jacket, which fell to the hardwood floor.
As I was being lowered, I pulled out a
banner that read: WELCOME CBS SPORTS.

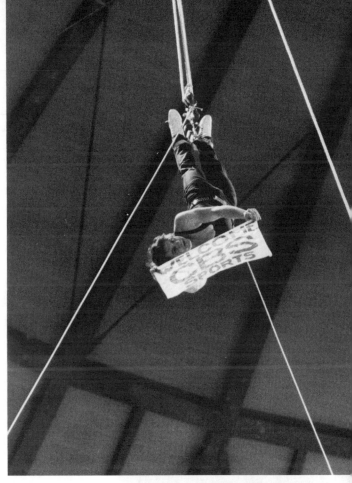

I really felt this was the greatest PR
moment of my career. I figured that
with the Pacers game on national TV, about five million
people had seen me do my escape. That's five million
seventeen thousand if you count the folks in the arena. Not
that I was counting.

Actually, I was about five million off. CBS had been
conducting a player interview during my escape, so the feat
never got on the air. The producer told me they'd taped the
event and would broadcast it later in the show.

It never happened. But I had still performed in front of the
biggest crowd of my career. And I loved every moment of it.

A few weeks later I would shift my focus from Pacers to
Racers, a team with the old World Hockey Association. A call
from their PR person led to my agreement to do a similar
promotional stunt at one of their period intermissions.

In a way this opportunity would result in a major shift in
how I performed escapes of this nature in the future. Because I
was concerned about my ankles (which had taken a beating
during previous stunts), I wore skates to negotiate the ice as we

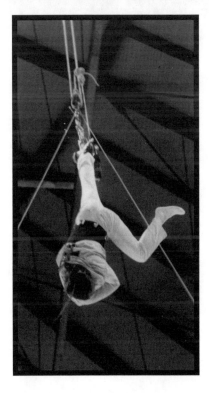

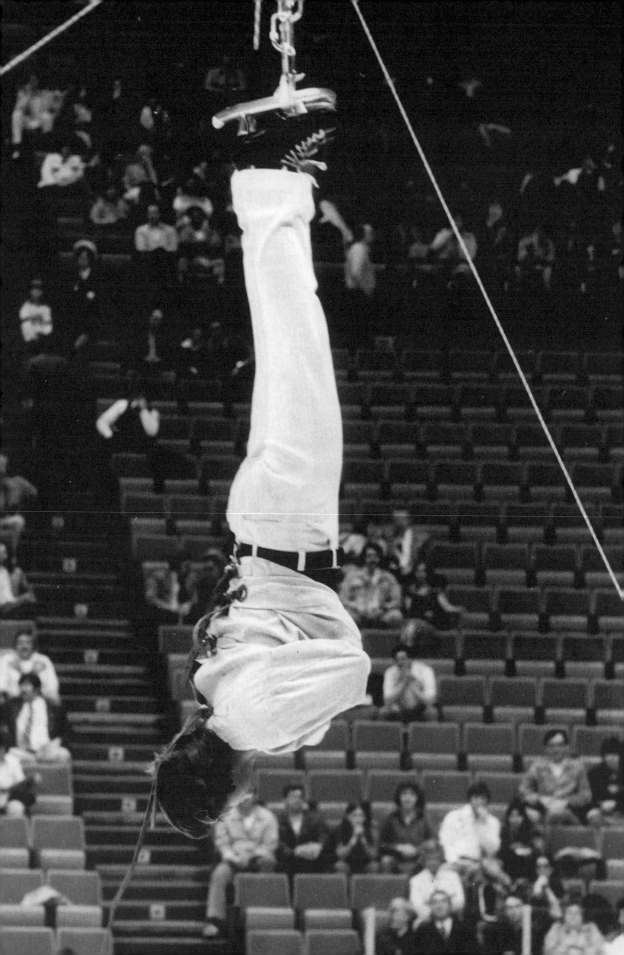

prepared for the event. I was a pretty good skater and felt I was less likely to fall on my butt during the preparations.

I had an idea. An idea that would not only be a benefit from a safety and technique standpoint, but tie the escape into hockey. I would hang from ice skates.

Spike Huber and I worked out the details, deciding that I would attach oval-shaped metal rings (mountaineers call them carabiners) to the blades and then directly to the pulley.

At the end of the first period, I skated with Racers captain Hugh Harris to the center of the arena. All I had to do was get in the straitjacket, clamp the rings to my skates, and have the crew hoist me upside down above the crowd. I was really loving this concept.

Shirk over ice. It had a nice sound to it.

Up, up I went. The hockey crowd, which I sensed would be harder to please than the basketball crowd, watched in stunned silence. I struggled furiously to free myself from the jacket. I wondered if a human looks different splattered on an ice floor than on a hardwood floor. Thoughts I should not have had.

Then came the surprise.

Prior to the event, I had loosened one of the skates. I had planned from the beginning to do the stunt hanging from just one ankle. I kicked the one skate off my left foot, and it dangled from the pulley. There was an audible gasp from the crowd. Was I halfway to falling?

I continued to struggle. The jacket came off. Once again, the restraint fell 100 feet to the floor, getting a bigger ovation every inch it fell.

Even when they lowered me to the ground, I was still on a high.

I went on to do other Pacer games, performing a double-burning rope, double-straitjacket escape, 50 feet in the air.

God, I love a crowd.

Up, up I went. The hockey crowd, which I sensed would be harder to please than the basketball crowd, watched in stunned silence.

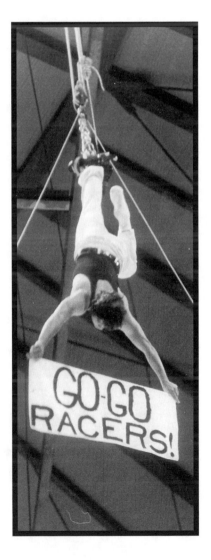

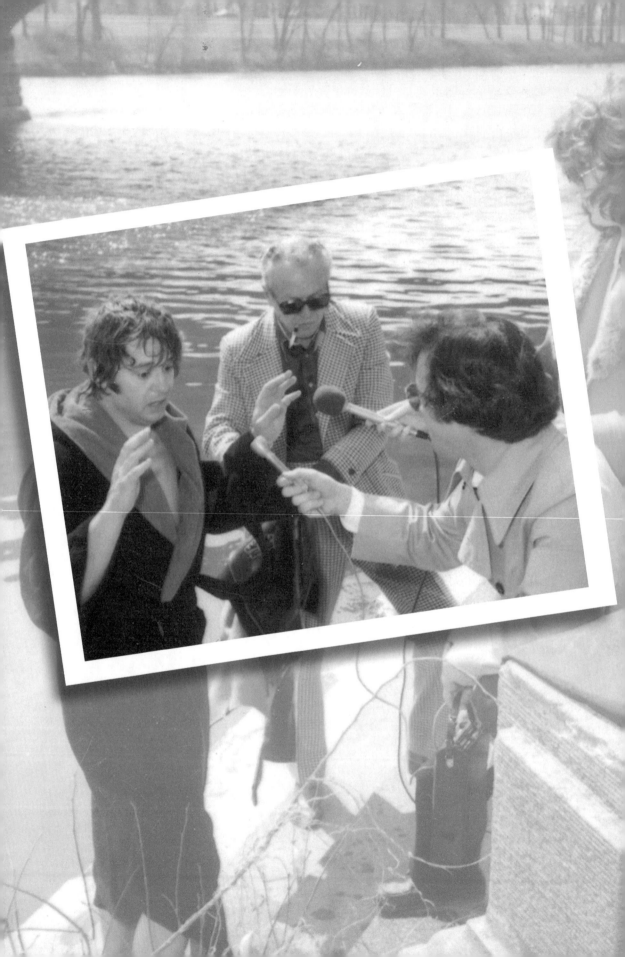

A Little White River Lie

IT WAS LATE MARCH 1978. Most Americans were gearing up to pay their taxes. Most radio jocks were looking for something funky to do on April Fools' Day.

April 1 is kind of a blank check in the radio business. It's the only day of the year you can do something totally deceptive and not worry about getting caught. If you *are* caught, you simply say: *It was a joke. April fool!* Don't try this on April 2. All the lawyers are listening again.

As a radio owner and promoter, I had been involved in my own share of shenanigans on April Fools' Day. A few years earlier we had intrigued listeners by playing the sound of a bouncing ball throughout the day. *"WXLW has balls,"* the announcer would bellow, and then urged people to call the request line. It was ultimately revealed, after we blew out half the phones in the city, that we were promoting a Pacers basketball game and were also giving away—what else?—basketballs.

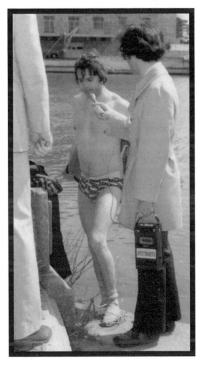

In another promotion I advertised in the newspaper for a wife—old hat nowadays, but pretty cutting edge in the late 1970s. Around the border of the ad, along with a dozen or so obligatory mentions that this was an advertisement (not news), was a sole reference to April Fools'.

Another favorite was my April Fools' announcement that a huge "something" had been seen swimming in the White River. We played tape recordings of people who claimed to have witnessed this behemoth in person. More than a hundred people showed up on April 1 to gaze upon the river in the hope of a "whale" sighting. No doubt these same people think they have been impregnated by aliens. (My ratings book never told me how many nuts were listening, just how many people.)

With a pretty good April 1 track record behind me, I was looking for still another promotion that would not only bring in some ratings, but land me on the front page of the local newspaper as well. In the past I had been relegated to the back pages, closer to the obits, where I am sure the newspaper people thought I would end up sooner rather than later.

Yes, April 1 was a perfect day for some daredevil escapade, plus my research on Harry Houdini had uncovered the fact that the master himself had been in the Circle City in April 1925. There he'd hung from the old *Indianapolis News* building and escaped from a straitjacket in front of 26,000 people.

My idea was to swim from the 86th Street Bridge in Indianapolis to the 30th Street Bridge, the same structure I had jumped off a year earlier. I promoted the White River swim as a 14-mile marathon, which was quite an exaggeration, but remember: *April fool*.

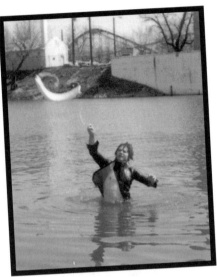

WXLW promoted my feat, but not until that very morning. We were not looking for a crowd when I left (and you'll see why), but we did want word spread that I would be making this ill-conceived swim, a trek that any clear-thinking person wouldn't do. In fact, any clear-thinking person would know it couldn't even be done.

Just like the Lone Ranger, you can't lead a life of danger without an assistant. My buddy Melvin Benn was my Tonto and, like Tonto, knew how to keep his mouth shut. What did he keep his mouth shut about? Read on, Kimosabe.

I entered the water at 6:00 A.M. dressed in a full wet suit and flippers. The water was frigid, barely above freezing, so numbing that within minutes of my immersion I could not feel any extremity of my body.

It would be an excruciating swim. Part swimming, part wading, part trudging through the shallow area of mud and rocks.

It would be an excruciating swim. Part swimming, part wading, part trudging through the shallow area of mud and rocks. Glass, old tires, garbage like you wouldn't believe. I knew if I made this, it would be a testimony to human endurance.

Five and a half hours later, I began the last mile. The thirty-eight-degree water had stiffened my body. My nose was gushing water and mucus. I was beyond feeling. I've never claimed to be a psychic, but I knew I was on my way to the hospital.

At one point two fishermen, themselves shivering on the shore, saw me making my way through the icy water.

"*Who are you?*" they shouted in unison.

I mustered all my strength to answer. "*Bill Shirk*," I trumpeted.

"*That figures*," came the orchestrated response. Hey, at least they knew who I was.

It had been six hours when I finally crawled onto the shore under the 30th Street Bridge and collapsed into some waiting arms. I'm not even sure whose arms they were. I do know that those arms wrapped a sorely needed warm robe around me.

Waiting for me were about twenty people, including an *Indianapolis News* photographer who snapped probably the most unflattering picture of me to date—a picture, by the way, that did end up on the front page of the newspaper.

I didn't talk to the media. I couldn't. I was shivering so badly, my teeth chattering so hard, that it would have been nothing but incoherent babble.

An ambulance arrived and I was whisked away to a round of applause from the small crowd. At the hospital I was diagnosed with pneumonia, multiple cuts and bruises, and a bad case of being out of my mind.

How does a human being muster the strength, the fortitude, the courage to swim in frigid water for six hours? How did I do it? The answer was simple:

I didn't.

How does a human being muster the strength, the fortitude, the courage to swim in frigid water for six hours? How did I do it? The answer was simple:

I didn't.

Having admitted all this now for the first time, make no mistake that I did enter the water as reported, but within five minutes I rounded a bend in the river and was out of sight. Then I simply swam to shore, where I got into a nice warm truck to wait out the morning. I read the paper, had some hot chocolate, and enjoyed a little classical music. And chatted with Tonto. I mean, Melvin.

It was then that I realized I could not negotiate the rest of the riverbed in flippers. I needed gym shoes. But gym shoes would not fit over the footies attached to the legs of the wet suit. So I took off the bottom half of the wet suit for the swim in.

Big, *big* mistake.

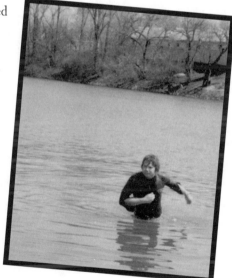

Five and a half hours later, I reentered the river near the bridge, again unseen by anyone. From about a mile out, I swam my way to the bridge, where I did suffer all the consequences reported above. That devastating effect on my body and the ensuing pneumonia were all the result of a mere thirty minutes in the water. Thirty minutes.

Did you think I actually made that entire 14-mile swim in six hours in a thirty-eight-degree river in half a wet suit and a pair of tennis shoes? You gotta be kidding. No one could have done that and survived.

Do you think I'm crazy? Not sure? You will be after you read the next chapter.

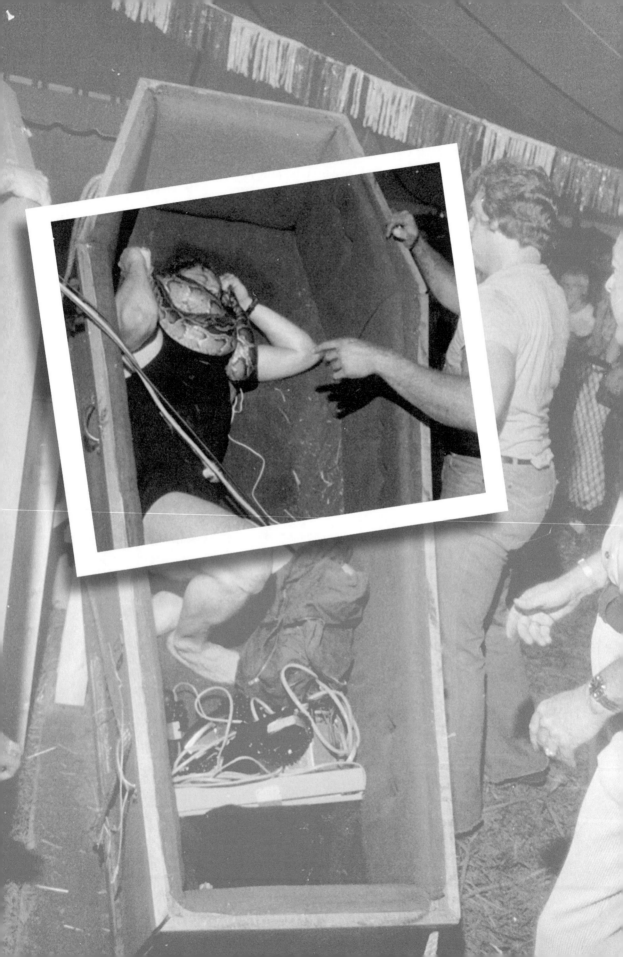

The Dirt on Burials

THIS WAS MY SECOND BURIAL, and you always feel that
the second time you do something it has to be even more
spectacular. The first time, I was buried for forty-eight hours—
no food, no water. I *did* raise $5,000 for charity, but it was not
the perfect escape. The coffin lid collapsed, we had an electrical
storm, and a 40-foot tent fell on top of me and knocked out the
air supply to the coffin. I was underground without electricity,
lights, or, for a while, air. Still, I felt I needed something else to
make this next escape even more exciting.

The answer was clear. I decided to share my space in the
oblong box with a few associates:
a 10-foot python, two tarantulas,
and a 5-foot rattlesnake. There's
nothing worse than being alone
in a casket, although come to
think of it you don't hear that
many complaints.

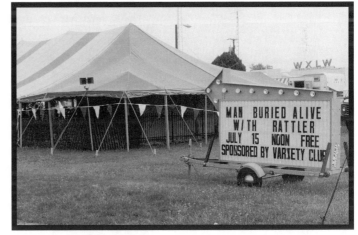

These kinds of escapes are far
more effective fund-raisers than
stuff like bridge jumps or
straitjackets because those are over
in minutes. A burial lasts several hours or days. People flock to
your location, and TV and radio people love it. In this scenario
I would hook up three phones and talk to media all over the
country—in fact, all over the world—twenty-four hours a day.
And at the burial site, hundreds of bystanders stayed and waited
for the outcome—and talked to me on the phone.

Publicity was my motive. That was what made Houdini
great. Not just his escapemanship, but his showmanship.
Houdini was the greatest marketer of himself who ever lived. I
liked that.

The first task was getting a coffin. I already knew this, so I
used my old coffin from the previous burial. Three and a half
feet wide, 3 1/2 feet high, 8 feet long. One room, no baths. Very
cozy.

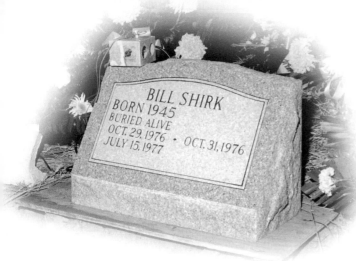

The next problem was finding someone who would loan me a 10-foot python. People who love pythons are very protective of their pets. They don't want their snake sleeping with just anyone. So I bought my own. I mean, if you're going to spend a few days and nights underground with a python, you want one that's friendly, sociable, and not apt to strangle or crush you to death. I have a publicity wish, not a death wish.

Two weeks before the escape, the snake died of pneumonia. I didn't even know a snake could get pneumonia. So now I was all set up for a big, live burial, but no snake. Don't you just hate it when that happens?

Dr. Jerry McVey, the Indianapolis Zoo veterinarian, suggested I talk to a local pet store manager, Larry Battson.

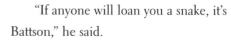

"If anyone will loan you a snake, it's Battson," he said.

I arranged to meet Battson, whose tiny bachelor apartment was home to every critter banned by his condominium by-laws. When I walked in the door the first time, Battson's girlfriend was standing on a chair screaming in horror, trying to avoid a slew of baby rattlers that had just been born. Boy did I find the right guy. I'm not sure his girlfriend felt that way.

His only python, named Crusher (great!), was a bit edgy. This meant he was nasty—nasty as hell. And he was a biter, which is a real danger with pythons, even though they are not poisonous. Pythons have tiny fishhook teeth. They can rip your flesh apart. You don't want to be bitten. But it is better than being crushed. (Not that you would ever have a choice.)

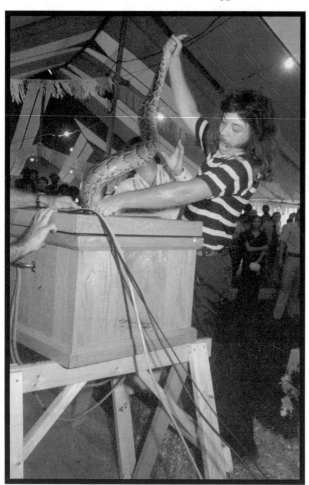

Ultimately Battson agreed to furnish me with everything: the python, the rattler, and the two tarantulas. I like convenience, so this was clearly the ultimate in one-stop shopping. The rattler, by the way, was the 5-foot timber variety. Maybe not the biggest in the world, but the biggest I ever saw. And, in fact, a record size for the state of Indiana. And very hot. That means poisonous.

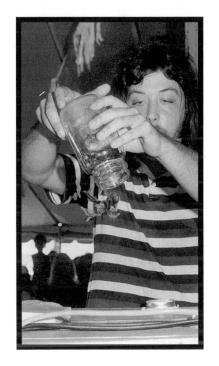

The day of the burial, it was eighty-five degrees, middle of July, and 1,000 people had come to watch the interment. I had on a long-sleeved jumpsuit, turtleneck, and sensible shoes. Underneath, I wore wrestler's tights. As soon as the lid was closed and sealed with me inside, I took off all my clothes, except the tights. That's harder than it seems. Try taking off your clothes while you're in bed without raising the sheets more than a few inches. That's about how much room I had. Plus it turned out to be a hundred degrees inside the coffin.

The animals were then inserted through a 1-foot-wide trapdoor in the lid of the wooden coffin. The two tarantulas were placed one by one through the trapdoor. I caught both in one of my shoes, then covered the shoe with my sock, tied a knot, and sealed it. The tarantulas were no longer a problem. Then the python slithered down into the coffin through the

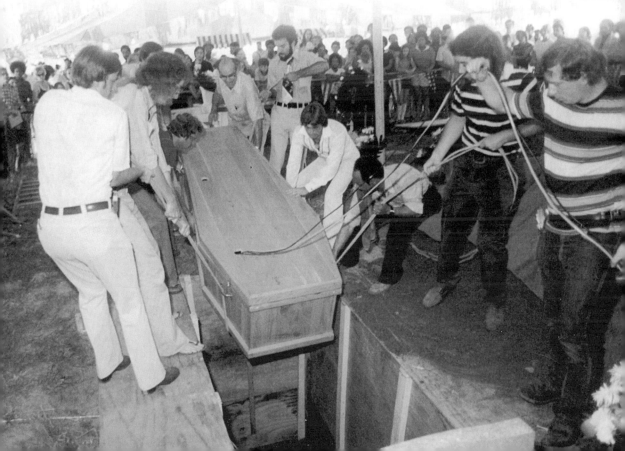

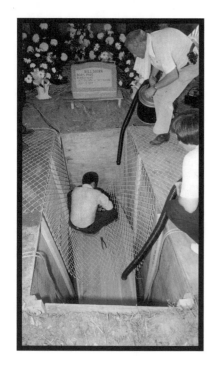

same door. I grabbed him (I think it was a him) by the back of the neck, put him inside my jumpsuit, tied both legs in a knot, and pulled the belt tight at the waistband. Now the python was pretty much contained. In fact, for the rest of the interment, I used the python as my pillow when sleeping and resting. I don't suggest this approach for folks with insomnia or people prone to bad dreams.

Then came the 5-foot timber rattlesnake. And this was the part I was having second thoughts about. In he wriggled through the trapdoor. I grabbed the rattler by the back of the neck, took one of my shoestrings and tied his mouth, then stuck him inside my turtleneck and sacked him up with the last shoestring.

I had not yet been buried, but the casket was shut so the folks at the burial site did not know I had effectively eliminated the risks posed by the snakes and tarantulas. Once again a vacuum cleaner was run in reverse and connected to the coffin. This was to be my only source of air.

The burial began. My coffin was slowly lowered into the ground. Then that first shovel of dirt. That's the scariest moment. It was a feeling that I can't describe. All the horror

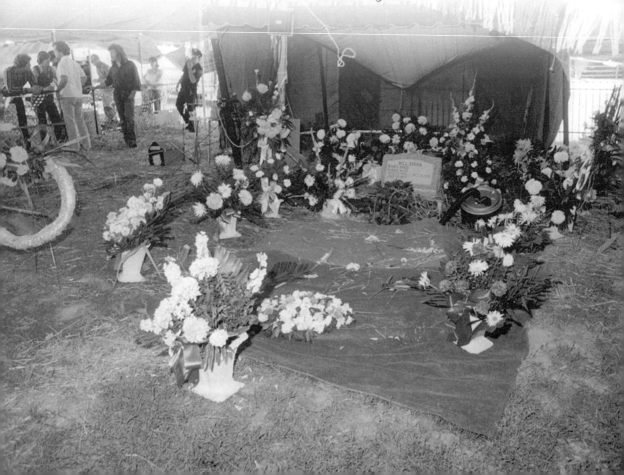

movies about coffins and live burials came back to me. I was lying there thinking, *This is every bad B movie I've ever seen.*

I wondered if the coffin would collapse again. Probably not. I had made sure that the box was supported by additional steel beams. Once again, this was just a working theory.

Remember, when I first did this burial stuff, I'd never thought I would actually stay underground for days. I had always envisioned a tunnel escape, so that while the world waited for me to be dug up, I'd be in an RV watching cable TV. Then I'd sneak back into the coffin.

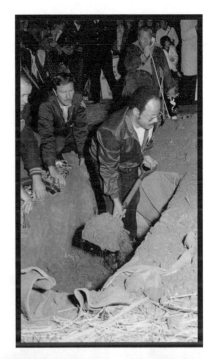

This is the way stunts like this are usually done. But this was for real. No tunnels, no RVs, no cable TV. Just me and my four closest friends. And those phones. Thank God for those phones.

After forty-eight hours underground, the money I had hoped to raise just never materialized. While hundreds stopped by the burial site, most of them giving money, I was still short of my goal. Frustrated, I told the world from 6 feet under that I would not come up unless President Jimmy Carter made a donation to my charity. The next day the *Washington Post* carried the story on the front page. By the time Carter's donation was received, I had spent seventy-nine hours underground—no food or water, but a lot of phone calls.

Just before I was dug out, I released the python and wrapped him around my neck. People assumed—and I can't help what people assume—the snake had been around my neck the whole time. Truth is, even in the few minutes the python was clutching my throat, I was gasping for breath and ready to pass out.

There were those who claimed the rattlesnake had been defanged or had its venom removed. When I climbed out of the coffin, Larry Battson took the

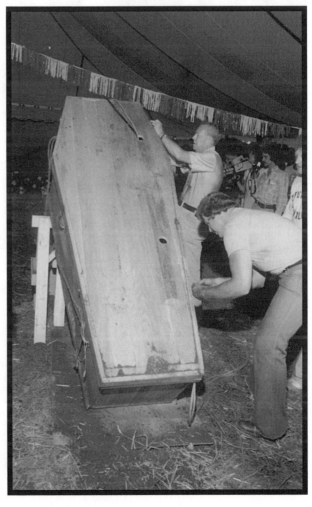

rattlesnake out of the turtleneck and milked it—putting the snake's mouth around a glass cup to show that venom leaked out. Proof positive that this snake was hot. I got a kick out of that. In some ways we had both milked the snake. Larry milked the venom; I milked the escape using the snake for everything it was worth.

Was I bored for three days underground? Never. Not for a second. I was on the phone all over the world, virtually every minute. I figure I did 200 interviews with radio and TV stations. I talked to hundreds of people who came to my burial site, waiting for me to "rise." I slept a few hours a night, usually between 3:00 and 5:00 A.M. Never a dull moment.

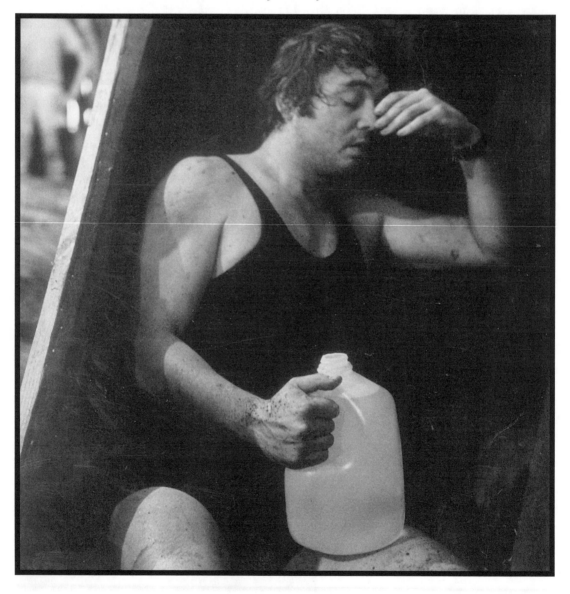

The most common question I am asked is what I did about going to the bathroom. I completely cleaned out my system before being buried, then, as before, I took Lomotil to plug myself up. I did urinate once or twice in a bottle. I'm telling you, that's the most common question. I think people have a greater fear of not finding a bathroom than being bitten by a 5-foot timber rattler.

In retrospect this was a pretty smart stunt. The rattler was the only real problem. If I had been bitten, I was quite possibly a goner. There was antivenin up top, but still, even with the antidote there is a 50 percent chance of dying.

Would I do a burial again? Maybe, but I promised I'd never use a rattler in an escape like this. (That's a promise I later broke.) After the escape someone stole my coffin. How low can you go?

By the way, Battson should have made a similar promise. Weeks later he was bitten by this very snake and spent a week in the hospital. Yeah, that snake was hot, all right.

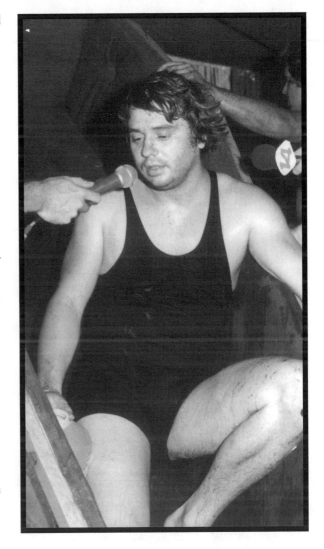

Would I do a burial again? Maybe, but I promised I'd never use a rattler in an escape like this. (That's a promise I later broke.) After the escape someone stole my coffin. How low can you go?

GUINNESS BOOK
-2-
WORLD RECORDS

IN 1 ESCAPE!

One for the Books

IF I'D HAD ANY SELF-DOUBTS at all at this point, it was not about my ability to do gutsy escapes, but whether I was approaching my goal to be the Number One Escape Artist in the World in the most efficient and effective way. True, my reputation had started to grow, but not as quickly as my ego, and I was still not officially recognized as anything except a little crazy.

I needed to do one for the books. Literally. And one book was the 1977 *Guinness Book of World Records*, a compendium of everything from the most hula-hoops spun around your waist at a time, to the fastest time to eat an entire bike, to Olympic records. If you were the fastest, longest, or highest, you were in the book. And sometimes the dumbest and

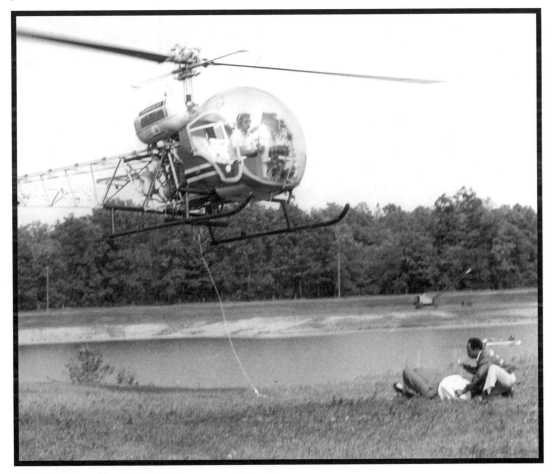

craziest made the book. That wasn't an official category, but I think you get the picture.

There were a few records listed under the general heading of "Escapology." All piqued my interest. All were beatable, including:

1. Highest escape from a straitjacket under a helicopter (1,200 feet), held by Paul Denver of Wales.
2. Fastest escape from a straitjacket standing on the ground (twenty-four seconds), by Herbie Becker, the Great Kerdeen.
3. Fastest jailbreak (five hours, fifty minutes), by Reynir Leossen of Iceland.

The records, especially numbers one and two, seemed at first glance pretty modest. I had already gotten out of a

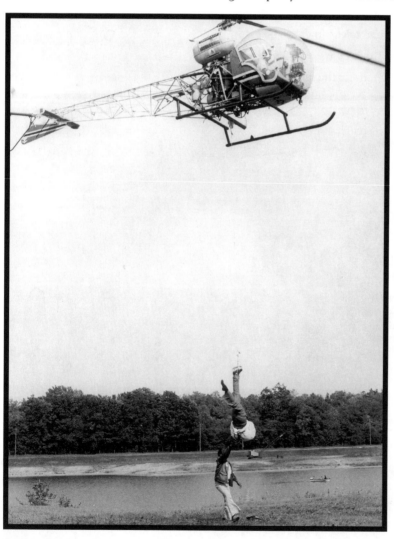

straitjacket in less than thirty seconds while hanging upside down at the wrestling match, and I had also freed myself 500 feet above the earth while hanging from my brother in Mexico. There was no reason I couldn't break both those records. At the same time.

By the way, Bob was happy there was no record for "longest time attached to your brother." He wasn't interested in breaking that one.

Now all I needed was a helicopter and a pilot. The Federal Aviation Administration informed me that any pilot willing to assist me in this endeavor would have to be certified to carry an external load beneath the chopper. I, of course, was the load and, according to my family, certifiable.

In past escapes I had managed to locate snakes, coffins, and bulls. I had gotten permission to jump off a bridge, convinced one guy to hoist me on a crane, and talked another into taking me parasailing. This time I needed a pilot willing to suspend me from his chopper in a straitjacket while I dangled from one ankle 1,200 feet in the air. This was not the assignment most serious pilots were looking for.

I'd like to think that it was my charm and wit that convinced a local pilot to assist me. It wasn't. It was $1,000, a fortune in 1977, but clearly a required stipend for a pilot to risk his reputation and career on an assignment of this nature.

Back to the FAA. They wanted to be sure that I wouldn't fall and kill someone else. That's right. I was expendable, but they didn't want some guy plummeting out of the sky and crushing a little old lady walking her toy poodle.

Once again, Frank Powell saved the day. Frank was sponsoring a picnic to raise money for the Marion County Association for Retarded Citizens. The picnic was to take place at a lake within the city. Doing the escape over water would reduce the chances of killing an innocent person. Of course, if I hit the water after falling 1,200 feet, I'd be catfish chow at the bottom of Lake St. Maur. Like I said, in 1977 the FAA didn't seem to care about that. They do now.

The basic elements of the escape were similar to the ones I had performed at the hockey game. I was going to wear a single skate and attach the blade to a cable, which would hang from the bottom of the chopper. I would then be suspended upside down during the escape. The problem was that I was going to be so high up, I would only be a speck in the sky. I could have been buck naked and no one would have known.

The helicopter's altimeter would be used to verify the height, a crucial detail if I wanted to get into the record books.

Now here's the big shocker. I actually practiced this feat. I suspended myself from my living room ceiling so I could practice upside down. I put up large fans to simulate the wind and cranked up the stereo to get used to the noise. I was still a

By the way, Bob was happy there was no record for "longest time attached to your brother." He wasn't interested in breaking that one.

bachelor then, and I'm sure any woman who saw the contraption I had set up would have made her own quick escape.

On August 1, just days before the scheduled flight, my pilot chickened out, concerned that my death could put a damper on his reputation. A mad search followed and I did find another pilot, Wayne McDermott, who had actual experience working with stuntmen in movies. In addition, he had been in Minnesota fighting forest fires and was used to carrying heavy loads of water beneath the aircraft to dump on the blaze. McDermott wanted $1,500 for the job.

Except for that part, he was perfect.

The day of the escape we met with the FAA inspector in person. Wayne brilliantly suggested that we both smoke cigars, which he believed would increase the chances that the inspector would want to speed up his investigation, especially if we puffed in his direction.

The idea seemed to work, but the inspector expressed concern that the chopper did not have a manual override, which basically meant that if there was an electronic malfunction, I would automatically be released—like the barrels of water to douse the fire.

To me the solution seemed simple: Couldn't we just attach a safety line to the landing gear of the helicopter? Not so fast. This was against regulations, and they wouldn't let me do it. That was decades ago and I still don't understand it. But no safety belt was allowed.

The day was overcast—not really a safety concern, but it did reduce the number of people at the picnic who could view my record-breaking attempt.

Assisting me in this endeavor was Marion County sheriff Don Gilman. His role was crucial, because Guinness records had to be witnessed and certified by some law enforcement agency. It was Gilman who also fastened the straitjacket on me, a jacket that was specially purchased for Guinness records so that each escape attempt could be fairly compared.

We attached a transistor radio underneath the jacket, then ran the wire up my back and attached an earpiece. The point here was to alert me when the timing of the escape would

On August 1, just days before the scheduled flight, my pilot chickened out, concerned that my death could put a damper on his reputation.

begin. *Dumb, dumb, dumb,* and you'll see why.

My associates were very busy. Wayne confirmed that the cables were attached securely to the chopper and the skate. Sheriff Gilman confirmed that the stopwatch was operating and my brother was standing by with binoculars. Brother Bob was in a pretty good mood. This escape was not going to disable his groin.

I lay on the ground, ready for the bird to take me up. Wayne took it up slowly to prevent the "bends," a similar effect to what divers experience when they quickly change the surrounding pressure. As with diving, the pressure would decrease as I rose.

Now, what would an escape be without some minor problems to make things interesting? First, the pain on my ankle was excruciating as the chopper rose. In retrospect (where I am always smarter), I should not have hung from one ankle. This did not have

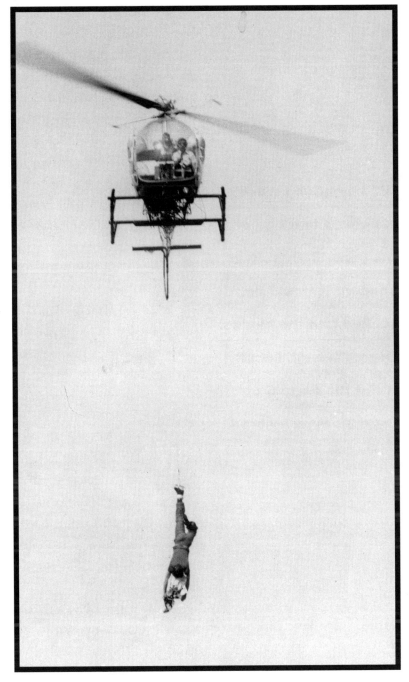

any record-breaking benefit, and people below could not tell the difference. This was a painful decision I had made. And it was the wrong one. As you may recall, this was the method I had used at Market Square Arena, where I hung by one skate at 100 feet for less than a minute. Big difference. Real big. This time it would be for fifteen minutes.

Here was another wrong decision. I should have been the one to decide when the straitjacket escape was to officially begin. Instead, I was dependent on a transistor radio that kept cutting in and out. Suddenly I realized that Paul Scheuring, the WXLW news director, was broadcasting the event live and had begun his countdown. I had already lost about eight seconds. It would be impossible to restart, so I frantically jerked the jacket over my head and let it drop.

Did I mention I wasn't supposed to let go of the jacket? There was concern it would be sucked into the blades. Oops. Oh well. Luckily it's at the bottom of Lake St. Maur instead.

Some good news. I had extricated myself from the straitjacket in record time, 22.5 seconds, and did it 1,610 feet above the ground, breaking the old records by 410 feet and almost 2 seconds.

It was a good thing I didn't pee in my pants because I had stuffed a banner in my trousers that I unfolded as we descended. It read: GUINNESS BOOK—2 WORLD RECORDS IN 1 ESCAPE!

Yes, it was true. The old record for a straitjacket had been 24 seconds, and that was on the ground.

It was over. And except for the excruciating pain in my ankle, I was pleased that I had not been in any real danger. At least, that's what I thought.

I was then informed by my pilot that the electronic hook release could have been activated by a stray radio signal from a CB radio. The bad news is, I would have dropped sixteen stories into the lake. The good news? I wouldn't have killed that toy poodle.

Yes, I thought I'd be in the *Guinness Book of World Records*. Twice. But I wanted to be in there three times. Three's a charm, they say. Or a hex.

The bad news was that someone already had broken one of those records. This came as quite a shock, but I learned that the time gap between when I broke the records and when the book was published each year had given me inaccurate information as to who the current record holders were. The

Did I mention I wasn't supposed to let go of the jacket? There was concern it would be sucked into the blades. Oops. Oh well. Luckily it's at the bottom of Lake St. Maur instead.

1978 edition, already at press, would show that Steven B. Burke had broken the straitjacket escape record on the ground with a time of ten seconds. I was already looking ahead to 1979.

My escape from a jacket 1,610 feet in the air was pretty spectacular, and remained a world record. There was, however, a new category: time to escape a straitjacket while hanging from the bottom of a helicopter hovering at 200 feet.

Yes, I was still the height champion, but I needed to capture those other three records for the 1979 edition, and I needed to do it all by that summer.

I had eight months. I wondered if my luck would ever run out.

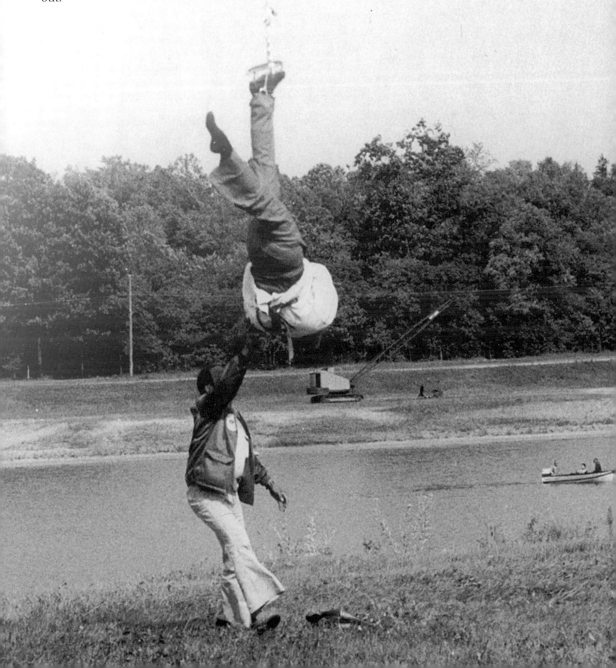

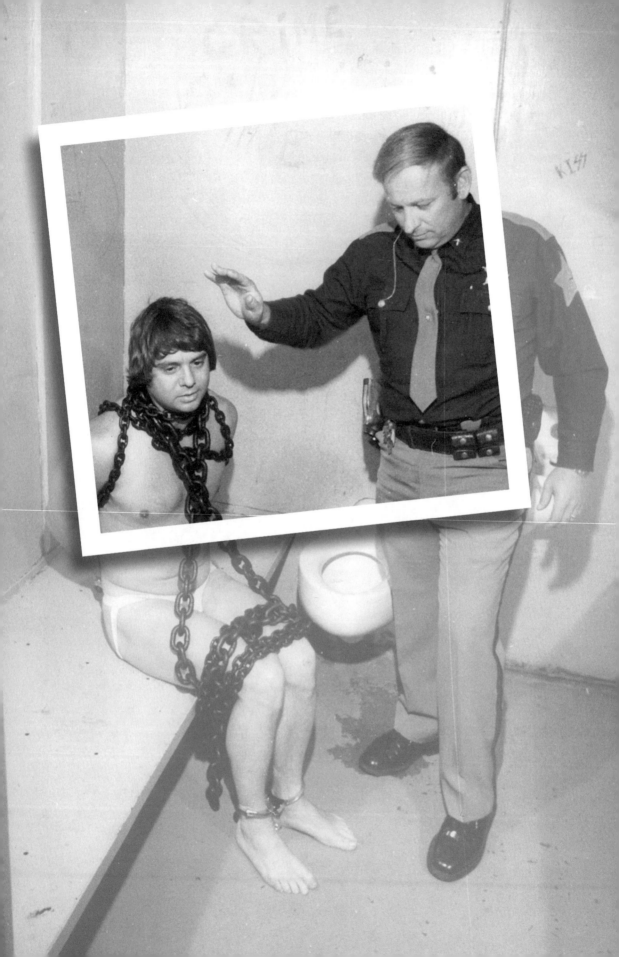

Fastest Jailbreak— Bar None

SOMETIMES PEOPLE ASK WHAT I MEAN by the word *escape*. Being buried alive was not technically an escape from anything; nor was running from the bulls in Spain really an escape. Unless, of course, you view the activity as escaping death. If that is the definition, then all the stories you've read so far are legitimate examples of escapes.

And of course, they were all successful—or I wouldn't be here today.

The word *escape* has always been linked with the word *jail* or *prison*. Countless books and movies chronicle daring and desperate, even reckless, attempts to attain freedom.

I always thought there was a certain poetry in the very phrase *prison escape*. And I had been thinking about trying my hand at one for a long time. I wanted to own that world record as well. But I also knew I was inexperienced in this area— and a failure in an endeavor like this could have terrible consequences for my career.

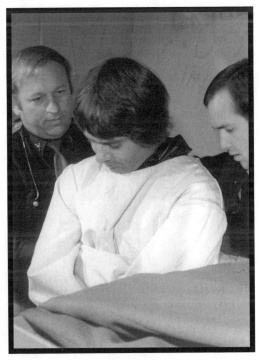

Escape artists get good publicity when they succeed. They get great publicity when they fail.

Finding someone who would let me jump off their cliff (see That Jumpy Feeling) or bridge (see Bridge Over Troubled Water) was easy compared to finding someone who would let me break out of their jail. Inherent in my request was my belief that I would be successful, which would result in the kind of publicity most law enforcement officials did not want for their institutions.

If I have been lucky in one area of my life, it's been my knack for meeting the right people at the right time. A phone call from a local magician and disc jockey Tom Ewing would start the wheels in motion for my second and third world records.

Tom was something of a student of the history of jailbreaks and confirmed for me that breaking out of a high-tech, modern-day facility was unlikely, if not impossible. He did, however, suggest that I look into the old jailhouse atop the Hamilton County Courthouse in Noblesville, Indiana. Because a new jail had been built, Sheriff Larry Cook was amenable, even tickled,

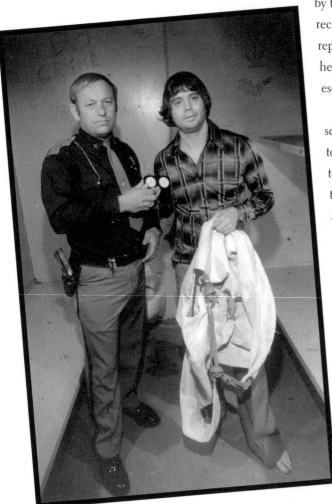

by the idea of being involved in my world-record quest. Although the old jail was being replaced, Cook had a special place in his heart for it. He even bragged, "No one has escaped from this jail in a hundred years."

Cook took this whole thing very seriously. He realized that the escape had to conform to Guinness's strict parameters to be counted. I would be locked with three pairs of handcuffs behind my back and have my hands tied by 5 mm chains, each able to withstand the force of 2,800 pounds. In addition, my feet would be fastened with footcuffs tethered with 5 and 10 mm chains with a tensile strength of 13,400 pounds and weighing 44 pounds.

Was this guy the sheriff or the county auditor? And what was I getting into? Or rather, what would I be getting out of?

Cook had also researched the current record—as I've mentioned, that was five hours, fifty minutes, by Icelander Reynir Oern Leossen. Leossen, I learned, was a strongman. I was only headstrong. But that would have to do.

I knew little about breaking out of jails except what I had read in my Houdini research. Houdini garnered massive publicity for a jail escape. I also consulted with a few prison inmates, kind of a funny approach because if they were so damn smart they wouldn't still be behind bars.

The key to Houdini's success (other than a key, as you'll see) was his knowledge of the different kinds of cuffs. Ewing collected cuffs, and we practiced at his house getting out of several versions, each time using a pick (a flat strip of metal or wire) to release the lock. And that wasn't the tough part of the escape. I still had the jail to deal with.

Taking a cue from Harry Houdini, I requested three visits to the jail under the guise of inspecting the environment. The sheriff was happy to oblige. He didn't know what I was really up to.

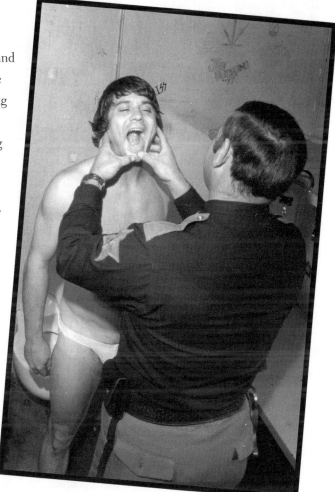

The first was truly a "get acquainted" visit. I observed the leg irons, handcuffs, and chains. There were two sets of bars on the door of the cell; outside the cell was a long corridor where, at the end, there was another solid steel door. This wasn't going to be easy.

My second visit was really the beginning of the escape. Just as in magic, where the trick really begins way before you think it does, the same is true of escapes. It was during this second visit that I requested proof that the old locks were still working. While the sheriff's deputy was fiddling with a number of keys, I managed to palm one of the duplicates in the confusion. In addition, I placed a small wooden wedge in the basement window of the jail, all in anticipation of my unscheduled return.

If this revelation disturbs you or bursts your bubble, remember that an escape is an illusion and that my role as an escape artist is to make good on my boast. "I can break out of your jail," I'd told the sheriff. Anything I did to make that happen was legit. The public just wanted to see if I could get out. When a guy makes a hole in one, you don't analyze his swing. You just go to the bar and celebrate.

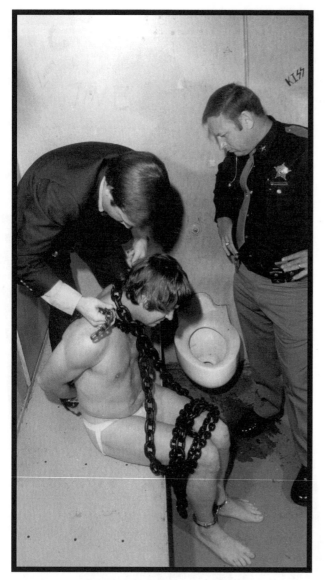

Before I was going to break out of the jail, I needed to break into it. At 3:30 A.M. on the day of the escape, Tom Ewing, my brother, Bob, and I actually broke into the courthouse through the rigged window and made our way to the jail cell. Using the duplicate key, we got inside, whereupon I used chewing gum to hide a wire and pick under the cell bed. Then we left the duplicate key on the ledge of the steel door down the corridor.

We arrived back at the jail at seven that morning. But before the jail escape, I had one more item on my agenda: the standing straitjacket record. Inside the open jail, with the assistance of the local sheriff, I was strapped into the strait-jacket. In a flash (4.92 seconds to be exact) I was free of the jacket and the official world record holder. I had beaten Steven B. Burke's record by more than five seconds. And I had done it using a technique taught to me by Tom Ewing. (See the sidebar on page 75.)

Back to the jail escape. I stripped down to an athletic supporter and allowed myself to be searched. The sheriff wanted to be sure that I had not concealed a key or pick on my person. Heh heh!

The morning was very cold, and I was shivering. A grown man shivering in his jockstrap and chains does not make a pretty picture. The sheriff and his deputies quickly put me in three pairs of handcuffs, leg cuffs, and chains; then they left after shutting both cell doors. I heard the door slam shut at the end of the corridor.

I went to work. The gum had literally frozen on the metal frame, making it almost impossible to free the pick. This was the last problem I had expected. I worked feverishly, which is exactly how I felt, finally freeing the pick and then manipulating it in each of the locks. The multiple restraints required all sorts of contortions on my part to position myself properly, but as I shed each one, the next became that much easier.

Now the double cell doors. I was totally spent, void of any energy to continue. Suddenly the proverbial second wind came. I found the sliver of wire in the second piece of gum and began work on the cell door. The first door opened quickly, but the second was older and more rusted. After twenty minutes of delicate maneuvering, it opened.

The corridor door opened easily with the key I had hidden on the ledge. It was here I found my discarded clothes and dressed.

One hour and thirty-seven minutes after my incarceration, I was free. Free to tell the world that I was getting closer and closer to being the Number One Escape Artist in the World. But where was the world? I was reveling in my success all alone. The very nature of this escape prohibited adoring fans from watching me. You don't want them to know about hidden keys. Illusion, remember.

I looked out the jail window and saw that a large crowd had gathered. The Houdini

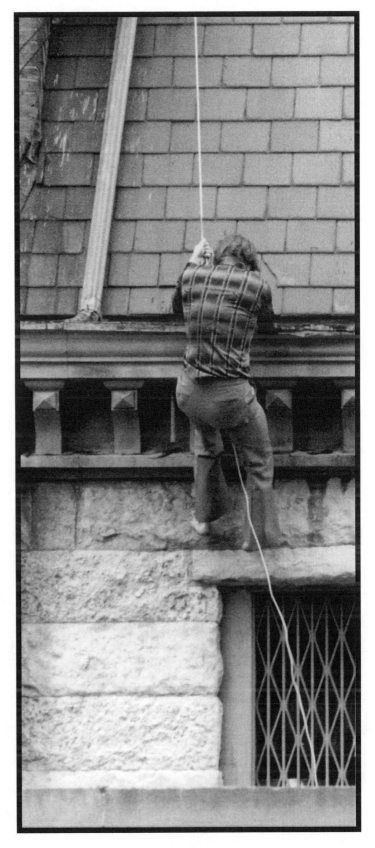

. . . Free to tell the world that I was getting closer and closer to being the Number One Escape Artist in the World. But where was the world? I was reveling in my success all alone.

showman was still in me. *Stretch it out!* I could hear Houdini say. After all, I had just broken the jail escape record by more than four hours. And I knew that breaking my own record in the future had PR possibilities. I was in no rush to depart the jail.

I sat tight for more than three hours. Then I grabbed a rope and rappelled down the side of the building to a cheering crowd.

Sheriff Cook was a good sport, congratulating me on my success. "Great job, Bill. Now how about trying to get out of the new jail?"

Not a chance. I had beaten the old jail escape record as well as the ten second straitjacket record and it was time to move on. I knew records were made to be broken. And others would be trying to break mine.

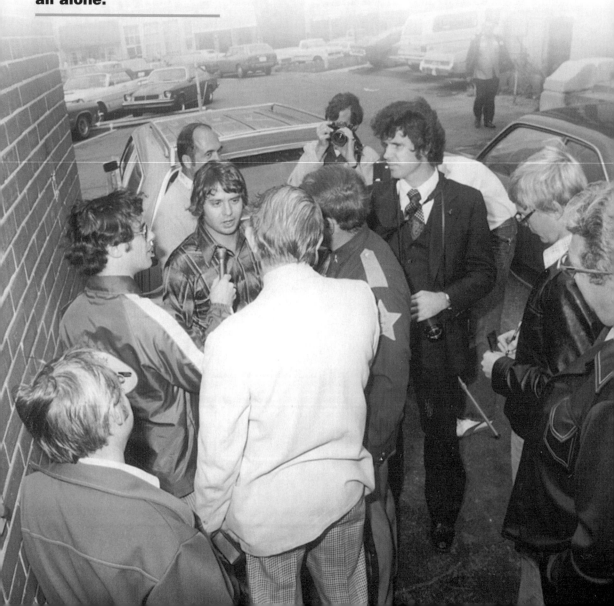

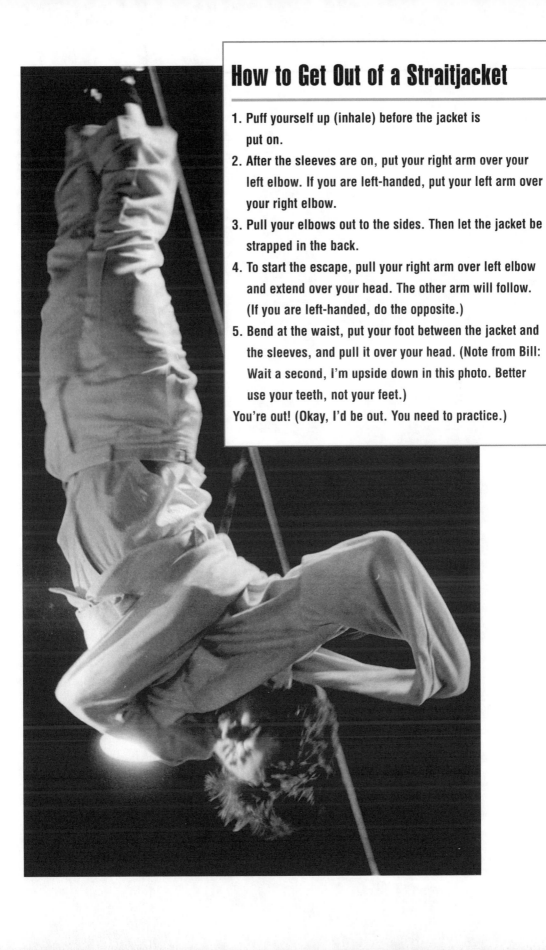

How to Get Out of a Straitjacket

1. Puff yourself up (inhale) before the jacket is
   put on.
2. After the sleeves are on, put your right arm over your
   left elbow. If you are left-handed, put your left arm over
   your right elbow.
3. Pull your elbows out to the sides. Then let the jacket be
   strapped in the back.
4. To start the escape, pull your right arm over left elbow
   and extend over your head. The other arm will follow.
   (If you are left-handed, do the opposite.)
5. Bend at the waist, put your foot between the jacket and
   the sleeves, and pull it over your head. (Note from Bill:
   Wait a second, I'm upside down in this photo. Better
   use your teeth, not your feet.)

You're out! (Okay, I'd be out. You need to practice.)

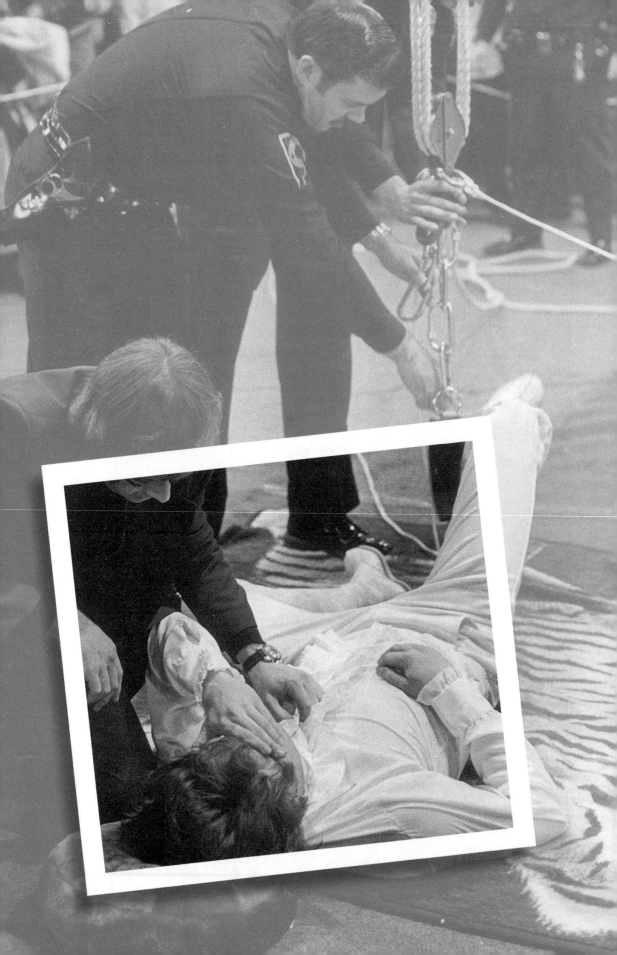

Auto Neurotic

SO WHERE WAS I THE WINTER OF 1978? I held three world records (so far). And I was getting some national—even international—publicity from a few of my escapes.

But my life had become a kind of vicious cycle. In a way, I couldn't win.

If I felt an escape was poorly planned, poorly executed, poorly attended, or poorly publicized, I was unhappy with myself. Usually things went pretty well, but then I was obsessed with finding a way to top each previous performance. How could I make the next escape better? Higher? Faster? Scarier?

In early December 1977 I got a call from the Indianapolis Auto Show, a huge event with a long tradition in Indy. To this day it remains a premier event, attracting tens of thousands of people eager to see the latest cars as well as the vehicles of the future.

Their offer to have me perform three times provided a unique opportunity. In my past escapes I had been pretty good at self-promotion on the radio. Heck, I owned the station. There was also a fair amount of pre-event publicity in the newspapers. But television news was not open to filling their precious time promoting some guy trying to kill himself, especially a guy who owned a radio station and competed for audience. They did, however, have lots of time for stories about guys who tried to kill other guys.

TV advertising can be bought, of course, but even in the late 1970s TV time was expensive, especially in comparison to the free promotion on radio and in print that I was getting. Inherent in the auto show deal was the opportunity to actually shoot commercials that would advertise my appearance at the

How could I make the next escape better? Higher? Faster? Scarier?

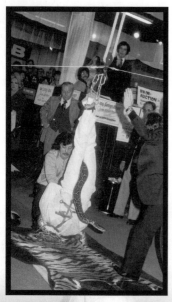
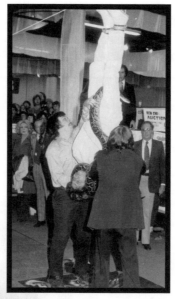
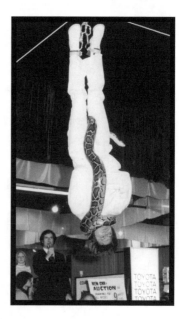

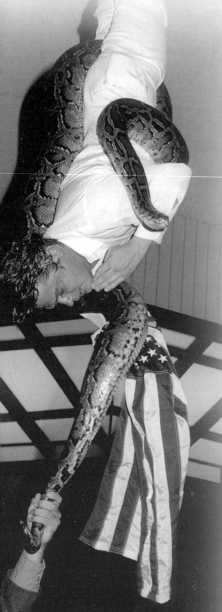

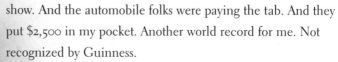

show. And the automobile folks were paying the tab. And they put $2,500 in my pocket. Another world record for me. Not recognized by Guinness.

The ads we did were a bit hokey. They featured me in a jail prying the "iron" bars apart as if they were huge Tootsie Rolls. The ad called me the Number One Escape Artist in the World and promised an exciting show if people came to see me perform.

The pressure was on for me to be spectacular, but I was soon to learn that I didn't have quite the venue that I'd had at Market Square. The show was at the state fairgrounds in the exposition hall, an old building with a very low ceiling.

It was from this ceiling that I had planned to suspend myself and do some kind of straitjacket escape while hanging upside down. This meant that when I was suspended, my head was only 15 feet from the floor.

I needed something to spice things up.

I called Larry Battson again, that local piece of work who was crazier than me. I was risking my life every couple of weeks, but Battson lived with poisonous snakes, reptiles, lions, crocodiles . . . you name it, and Battson had been bitten by it. He used the animals to educate local schoolkids, but I swear he tested them on himself first to make sure they were safe.

Battson suggested that to make the escape more dramatic, I should drape his new 10-foot Burmese python around my neck and body as I hung, upside down, from my heels. He was still hyped up about the burial extraction, proud of the role his snakes had played. Battson was sure the snake was docile and not a biter, but I still thought he was giving the reptile a final test with me before he let a six-year-old play with it.

The first day of the show, I was surprised to see how close to the ground I would appear to the crowd. Falling 15 feet onto cement is very dangerous, but it didn't have the same dramatic appeal as falling 1,600 feet from a helicopter.

Escape artists often fantasize what the headlines will be after a botched effort:

SHIRK KILLED BY MARAUDING BULLS
SHIRK FALLS 1,600 FEET FROM HELICOPTER
SHIRK DIES FROM RATTLESNAKE BITE

This escape did not have quite that potential for compelling reading:

SHIRK FALLS, BUMPS HEAD

Thank God for the snake.

The show began. First I was strapped into the straitjacket, then hung upside down by my ankles. Battson stepped up with a huge snake and gently draped him through my legs. I was hoisted 15 feet into the air. I am going to assume that most people reading this paragraph have not had a hundred-pound Burmese python in their crotch. If you have, you can skip this chapter.

While I wasn't happy about a reptile lounging in my crotch, the alternative was for him to wrap himself (or herself—who cares?) around my entire body and then tighten up so he wouldn't fall. I would be his tree. No thanks.

The escape began. I was hoisted into the air and started wiggling, fully aware that the snake's response to my gyrations was somewhat unpredictable. Plus if I moved too much, the snake would fall off and ruin the escape—*or* he'd wrap himself around me and constrict, and that would ruin me. I'd be choked to death.

The crowd was very excited, which apparently agitated the snake, whose tail was curled over my face. Then the snake peed in my mouth. Battson was laughing. This was the kind of

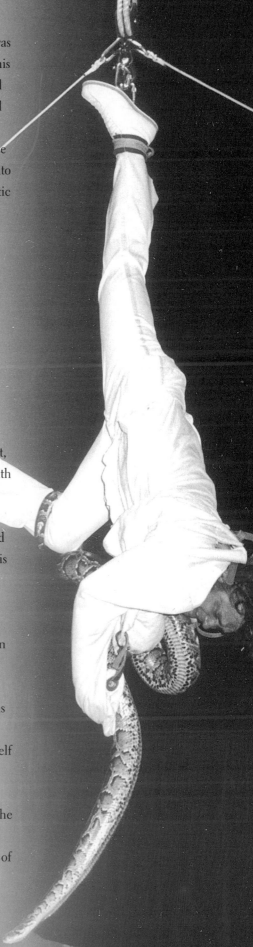

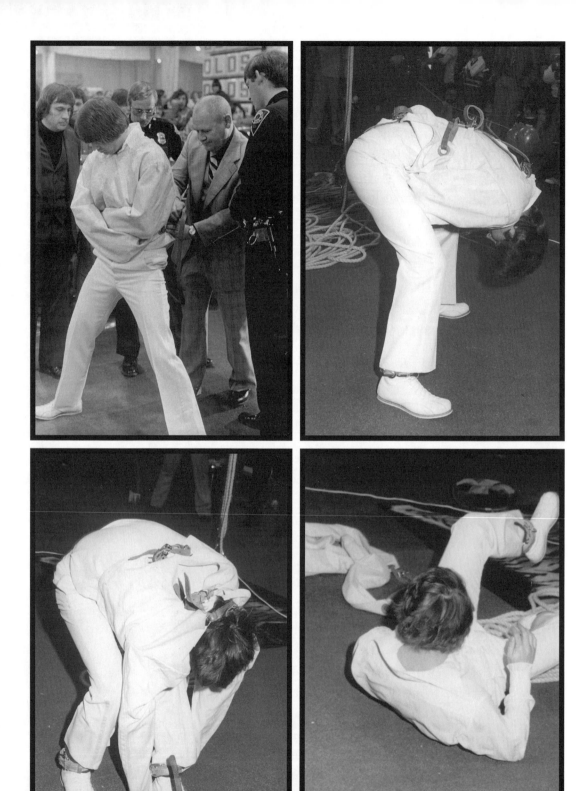

sophisticated humor that Larry loved. I made him promise that the next time we did this, he'd take the snake for a walk (crawl?) before we went on stage.

To spice things up during the second show, I slipped my foot out of the harness during the escape so I was suspended by only one ankle. This caused the anticipated gasp from the crowd. I shed the jacket, the snake fell into Battson's snake-loving arms, and I revealed an American flag that I had hidden in my shirt.

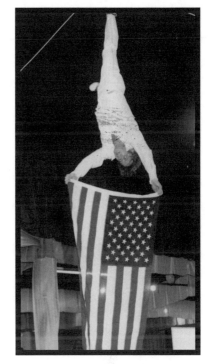

Then an inspiration. I decided on the spur of the moment to break my existing straitjacket escape record of 4.92 seconds. I was sure I could do it, in part because of the new method I had adopted with the advice of Tom Ewing.

Jim Wells, a lieutenant in the sheriff's department, was nearby and offered to strap me in and time me. His participation was crucial to verify and legitimize the escape for Guinness.

In the time it just took you to read the last sentence, the jacket was off. Total time: 4.52 seconds. I had shattered my own record. Okay, I didn't shatter it. But I broke it. And I had done it with snake pee in my mouth. Which, by the way, is not something Guinness required.

I went home very pleased with myself. Brushed my teeth about eleven times and started thinking about my third performance.

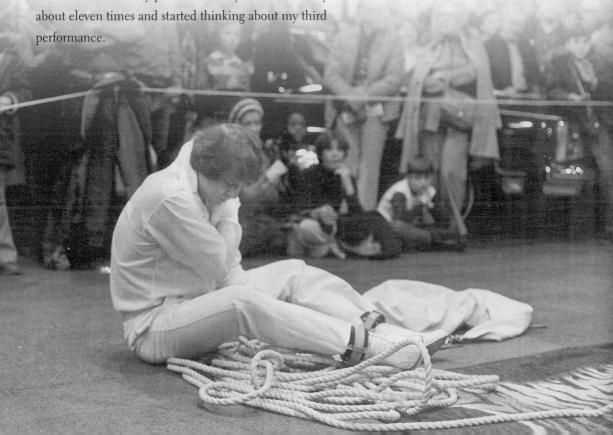

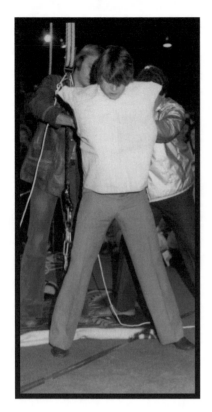

Actually I had been thinking about and planning this escape for several months. I wanted to hang from a rope while chained and handcuffed and get out of the restraints in full view of the audience. Let's see, I forgot to mention one detail: I wanted the rope to be on fire. I would complete the escape and be lowered to the floor before the rope snapped and sent me south.

Plans for the escape had started in an old warehouse months earlier, where I suspended 200-pound sandbags from various types of rope that I had doused in kerosene. I lit each rope and then timed how long it took for the bags (my weight) to break it. If I found that the rope would hold the weight for four minutes, I'd know my escape needed to be accomplished in two, giving me a safe margin of error. I also knew that the necessary contortions to get out of any restraints would effectively make the load "heavier."

The third performance began. A sheriff's deputy secured the cuffs and chains. I was hoisted upside down as a 5-foot section of the rope just above me was set on fire. The kerosene began dripping down from the rope onto my pants and shoes, and I feared my clothing would catch on fire. Not something I had planned on, but it would have gotten a big reaction from the crowd.

The third performance began. A sheriff's deputy secured the cuffs and chains. I was hoisted upside down as a 5-foot section of the rope just above me was set on fire.

My biggest concern at this point was getting the pick out of the plastic fake thumb on my left hand. Once I secured the pick, I feared dropping the tiny piece of metal and ending any chance I had to escape the restraints.

I began turning and gyrating, negotiating the lock. Some of the audience may have sensed what I was doing, but most were probably mesmerized by the fire. Once the cuffs were off and my hands free, the chains simply needed to be unwound. I signaled the crew to lower me. Total time, about two minutes, a pretty safe margin, but I had announced to the crowd that I only had two minutes. They thought I was seconds from death.

The auto show was a success garnering the largest crowd in its history. I was obsessed with what would come next. As far as I knew (there was no Internet in those days) I now owned three records:

1. Time escaping from a straitjacket on the ground.
2. Jailbreak escape.
3. Height hanging from a helicopter escaping from a straitjacket.

I wanted a fourth record. I more than wanted it; I was consumed by it. Why? I was convinced that by attaining a fourth world record and ending up in the *Guinness Book* for 1979 I would hit the mother lode. This would be my entree into fame and money.

The record I wanted was a new one in the 1978 edition recently conceived by the Guinness people. Jimmy Dixon of Florida had set a straitjacket escape record in Las Vegas while hanging from a hovering helicopter at 200 feet, getting out of the restraint in 19.9 seconds.

I had already hung from 1,610 feet, but this was a new official category at only 200 feet. I wanted that record. And I wanted it now. Well, not quite *now*, as you'll see in the next chapter.

I was convinced that by attaining a fourth world record and ending up in the Guinness Book for 1979 I would hit the mother lode.

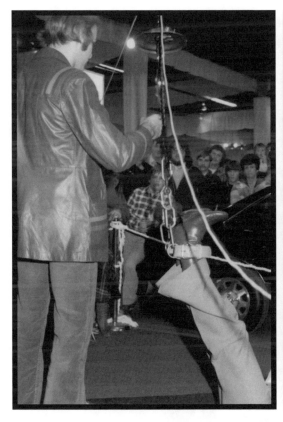
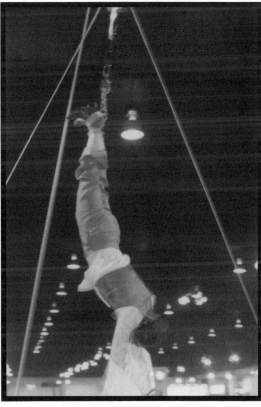

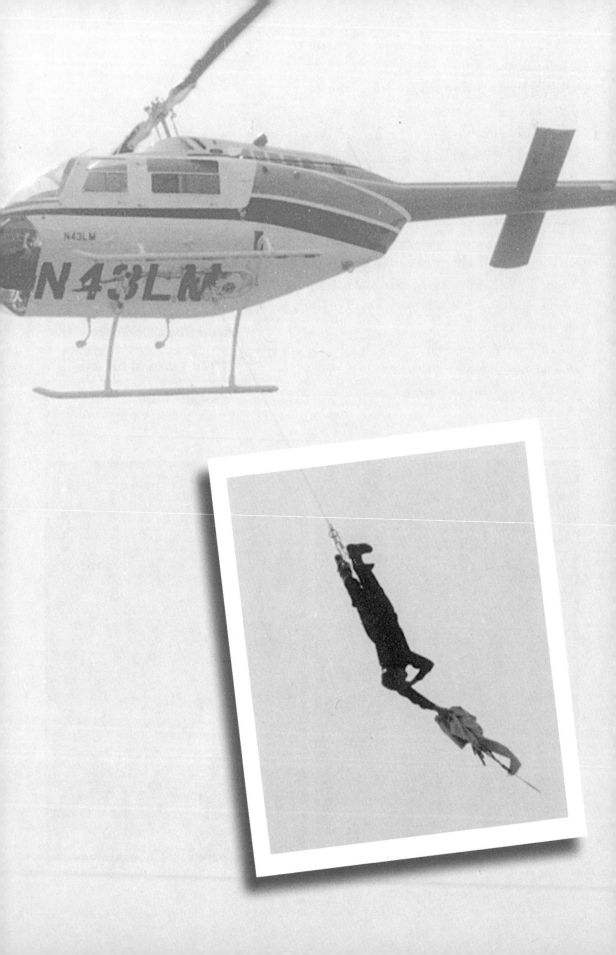

End of My Rope

I WANTED TO BE RICH. I wanted to be famous. There was only one way to do it: be the World's Number One Escape Artist. I wasn't going to get wealthy by owning a radio station. Ironically, I was wrong about that, as you'll see.

I had convinced myself that I was on the verge of attaining all my goals, but I faced one immediate challenge. I needed to hold all four Guinness escape records when the new 1979 edition came out in October 1978. If I could make that happen, I'd be set. For life.

I felt my other three world records were pretty safe. At least temporarily. I had confirmed with the Guinness people that my straitjacket record on the ground, my jailbreak record, and my 1,610-foot escape from beneath a helicopter had not been bettered. Generally, potential competitors will check with Guinness before making a record-breaking attempt to ensure that everything is done according to standard. No inquiries had been made regarding Dixon's record. That was good news.

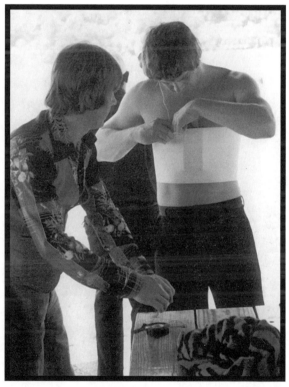

I further ensured recognition in the new edition by planning my helicopter escape toward the end of June, knowing full well that any pretenders to my throne would not have the time to set in motion an escape that was so complicated to orchestrate.

I had a lot of red tape to deal with, but first and foremost I knew that this escape required top conditioning. I hit the gym several times a week. Pumping iron and jogging—an exercise program with no direction. Even my jogging was on a circular track. I was getting nowhere . . . fast.

Once again I had gone a bit headstrong into a plan without enough thought. Fortunately, one of the trainers at the

There it was: Ideal Helicopter, in Wabash, Indiana. Not only were they willing to assist me with the escape, they were actually a little miffed I hadn't called them last time.

gym, Bobby Higgins, a former world weight-lifting champion, pointed out that I was wasting time in some of these activities. "You don't want muscles," he lectured me, "you want flexibility." Being the already flexible guy that I am, I took his advice. I began a regimen of stretching that included yoga, isometrics, and racquetball for conditioning.

My pilot from the last chopper escape was not available. I was so desperate that I had looked in the Yellow Pages. There it was: Ideal Helicopter, in Wabash, Indiana. Not only were they willing to assist me with the escape, they were actually a little miffed I hadn't called them last time. And, they personally knew the guy from the FAA who'd certified me back in August '77. Go figure.

My buddy Frank Powell again coordinated the PR effort, his promotions noting that the event would benefit a charity

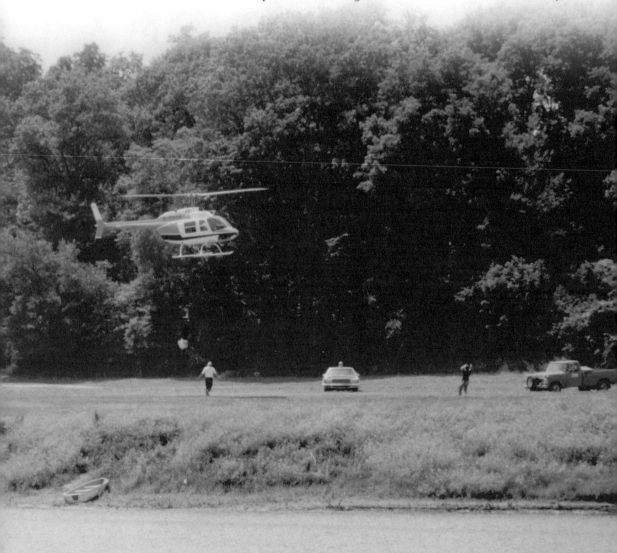

through Variety Club Tent 10. Powell also arranged for the escape to take place over Lake St. Maur, the same lake where I had performed my first helicopter escape. Remember, this time there was really something to promote. At 200 feet people could see what was happening. I would be more than a speck in the sky.

Everything seemed to be going as planned. In the grand style of Houdini, I also arranged for the Indianapolis police chief, Eugene Gallagher, to officially challenge me to get out of the straitjacket that he, personally, would strap on me. Houdini knew that such challenges increased the hype prior to the event, but at the same time gave the escape a certain credibility.

Publicity for the event was huge. My own station pumped it to death. Local papers and even TV seemed more intrigued with this one than some of the others. I was thrilled, but also very stressed—probably more stressed prior to this escape than any before. I had convinced myself that the stakes were huge and that failure was unacceptable.

And there was more stress to come. Lots more.

I got a letter from my friend Tom Ewing, who informed me that there had been a recent attempt by an escape artist in England to do a straitjacket escape hanging from a cable 22 feet below a helicopter, a distance I considered more than safe. But a gust of wind had rocked the chopper to its side. His weight acted like a pendulum, keeping him in a fixed position as the blades rotated and—I'm not sure how to say this politely—cut off his head.

This was not the kind of news you want the day before an escape. It would, however, probably fit loosely into the category "News You Can Use." Not that I did. I decided to keep the cable 12 feet long.

The day of the event, we had more problems with my buddy from the FAA. I'll never know for sure, but I still think he remembered how the last time, the pilot had blown cigar smoke in his face in an attempt to quicken his decision. Just as the smoke had lingered in his face, so had his hang-up over me as an external load under the helicopter. For reasons that to this day elude me, this bureaucrat refused to allow my pilot

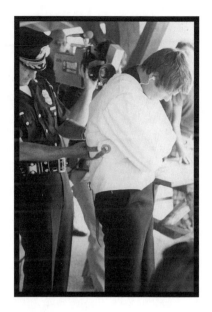

Everything seemed to

be going as planned.

In the grand style of

Houdini, I also arranged

for the Indianapolis

police chief, Eugene

Gallagher, to officially

challenge me to get

out of the straitjacket

that he, personally,

would strap on me.

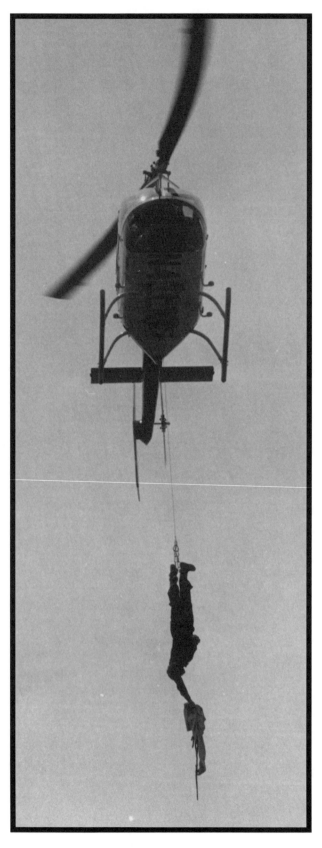

to use his manual override. Translation: Once again, I could be ejected from the bottom of the chopper due to some electrical malfunction or interfering CB signal. There was no fail-safe.

His reasons were never clear. They didn't have to be. That was the situation and I'd have to live with it. (Or die with it.) Oh well, the worst that could happen would be a 200-foot drop into the lake—the result being a few broken ribs, but certainly safer than hitting an ice rink or hardwood floor, or falling from 1,610 feet, three possibilities I had faced in the past year or so.

It was a beautiful day, not a cloud in the sky, but at 200 feet it wouldn't matter too much, anyway. I arrived in a limo, an entrance that always attracted attention, and greeted more than 1,000 people who had come to watch. It was a great crowd, but my approach to this escape was all business. Do it. Go home. Wake up famous.

A transistor radio was strapped to my chest so I could hear my own news team broadcast the event to the public. But more importantly, the radio would tell me when the timing would begin. This is the method that failed the last time at 1,610 feet, but this time I'd be close enough to the ground to provide better reception, plus I could actually hear the loudspeakers that would herald the beginning of the official time.

Gallagher strapped me into the jacket. Ultimately I would hang about 12 feet beneath the chopper. I slowly rose to 200 feet. The sound of the blades was almost hypnotic. I felt as though I were in a vacuum, and as I gazed up at the blades, they seemed to spin in slow motion. It was like being in a movie and experiencing the visual effects personally.

The chopper lurched. It jerked. It rocked. By the time that movement filtered down the cable to me, it felt as though I was about to be ejected from the bottom of the helicopter. For the first time I wondered if tomorrow morning I might wake up dead instead of famous. The thought didn't last long, but it did cross my mind. The time to beat was 19.9 seconds.

Five, four, three, two, one . . . GO!

And 18.83 seconds later, the jacket was off.

I could have literally popped off the jacket and made a better time, but even in my heightened state (excuse the pun), I realized that I did not want to shatter the record, just break it. I knew it was too late in the year for someone to better my time and envisioned myself breaking my own record on national TV. Man, was I flying high.

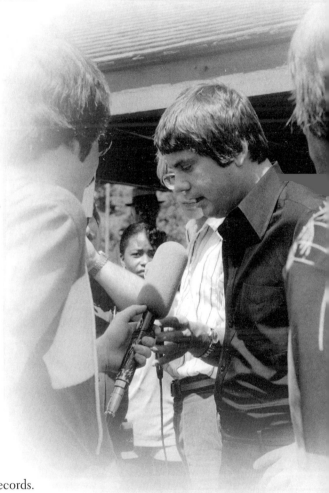

Minutes later, the chopper returned me to earth. I talked briefly to the media, but spent much less time with them than I had in the past.

As with all the escapes, there had been nothing enjoyable about it. If you have some grand vision about soaring like a bird under a helicopter, you need a fantasy readjustment. This was not fun.

It was all business. It was all about me. And now it was all over. I went home to bed. I wasn't sure I'd wake up rich and famous quite yet, but I figured I'd wake up with four world records.

And so I did.

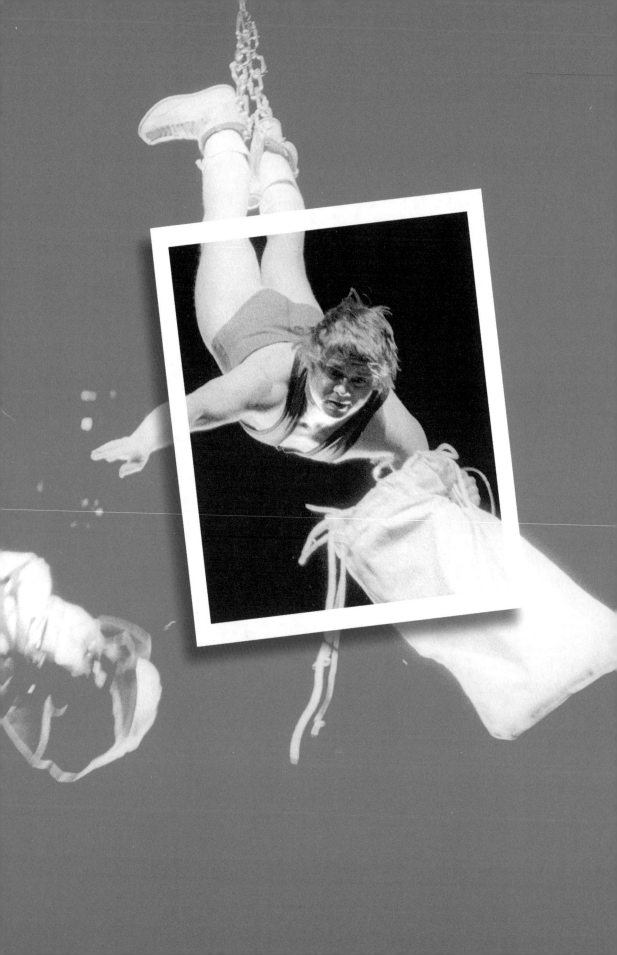

It's in the Bag

"YOU WANT ME TO DO WHAT?" I stammered during my breakfast meeting with Cecil Byrne, longtime booking agent for the Shrine Circus.

"You're not hard of hearing, are you, Shirk? Pay attention. I want you to hang by a trapeze, which will be attached beneath a motorcycle that will be traveling across a tightrope. And while you're doing that, you can get out of a straitjacket."

"Say that again!" I was incredulous. For the first time in my career I wasn't calling the shots. Someone else was telling me what he wanted me to do. And that someone was not just anyone, it was Cecil Byrne, a legend in the circus business and a man who had probably booked 1,000 acts.

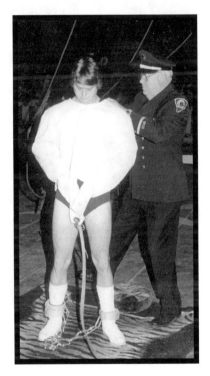

Byrne had seen it all, so the fact that he was interested in my performing center ring at the country's number two circus (second only to Ringling Brothers) was very flattering and career enhancing. Circus performers are a step above carnival acts, so an opportunity like this would provide a much-needed boost to my résumé.

Still, I was reluctant to accept the challenge. I had tried hanging trapeze-style in the gymnasium, but the pain in the back of my knees was so excruciating that I couldn't hold on for more than forty-five seconds. I know that seems odd coming from a guy who hung from one ankle under a helicopter for fifteen minutes, but I knew my body and it would not be happy with this. Don't believe it's painful? You try it.

I told Cecil I'd consider it, knowing the chances were small I'd accept the challenge. A couple of days later, the phone rang. Cecil informed me that the motorcycle act would not be able to make the circus and we'd have to come up with a new idea.

"Gee, what a shame," I said. I tried to sound like I meant it.

"Don't worry," said Cecil. "I have a better idea. You can hang in a straitjacket from a trapeze over a cage filled with lions and tigers."

"You want me to do what?"

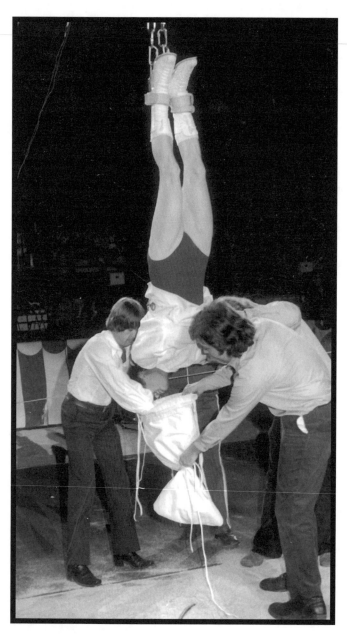

My hearing seemed to be getting worse. I gently refused, promising that I would come up with something spectacular for the Shrine Circus. I just needed a few days to think about it.

"It's got to be huge," grumbled Cecil. "And none of that burning rope stuff. I want BIG, BIG, BIG."

I went home and decided to call the only person I knew who was crazier than me. You guessed it: animal trainer and educator Larry Battson.

Battson was in love at the time. Not with a woman, but with a 6-foot eastern diamondback rattlesnake with 1/2-inch fangs and probably the deadliest venom in North America.

"This snake is a sweetheart," said Battson, "and he's our ticket to your fame and fortune."

"How's that?" I asked, afraid I would hate the answer.

"We're going to hang you upside down from the circus ceiling in a straitjacket and stuff your head in a bag with this snake."

"Say what?"

"Trust me, Bill. This snake is a lover, not a biter. Not to worry."

But worry is a good thing for escape artists. You need to worry about every escape, take nothing for granted, and plan every detail. This was uncharted territory. I had serious doubts.

I suggested to Larry that we sew the snake's mouth shut. Or maybe de-venom the reptile.

"Not my snake," he told me. "Not that adorable snake."

And so it was. I agreed to pose the idea to Cecil Byrne, hoping he'd think this was BIG, BIG, BIG. I called him on the phone the next day and told him my idea. "You are crazy," he said. This from a man who had booked some of the most dangerous circus acts known to humankind.

I also told Cecil that the snake was hot, meaning that it was fully capable of striking and killing, and that we would offer a $10,000 reward to anyone who could prove otherwise.

Cecil loved it. I knew he would.

There was no reason to practice this. What's to practice? Any idiot can put his head in a bag with a rattlesnake. I was just the first person to take the job. And I had to do it nine times over a four-day period.

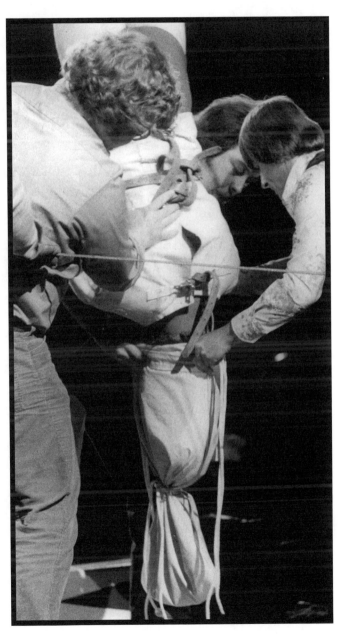

I was privileged each day to walk around the arena during the traditional opening of the Shrine Circus. That's when all the circus performers parade in front of the crowd so everyone in the audience can see close up who will be entertaining them.

I was very conscious of this honor, knowing that I would be seen, maybe for the first time, not as just an escape artist, but a true professional. That bubble was burst on the first day, when I stepped into about four pounds of elephant droppings in front of 14,000 people. It was the first time I really wished my head were already in the bag with a rattlesnake.

I was to perform after the first intermission. The announcer explained to the crowd what I was going to do and reinforced that I was the World's Number One Escape Artist. Many already knew about the nature of the act from the pre-event publicity, but there was an audible gasp when they heard it explained again over the loudspeaker. Even I was thinking: *Is that me he's talking about?*

Then Battson came out and held the 6-foot sweetheart up to the crowd. It rattled. The crowd gasped again.

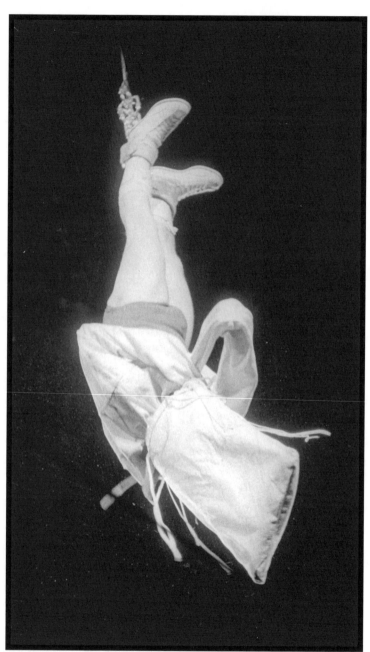

The straitjacket had been placed on me prior to the event to save time. I would be attached to an electric winch that would ultimately zoom me 100 feet in the air in a matter of seconds. The cable was attached to both my ankles, and the winch lifted me upside down about 2 feet off the ground. Then Battson placed the snake in the bag. The crowd was quiet now.

Battson held the bag under my head, opened it just wide enough, and slowly, very slowly, lifted the bag around my head. I think in all my hundreds of escapes, I have never felt so many people so uncomfortable with what I was about to do.

Battson tied the bag around my neck, and the winch lifted me almost 100 feet to the top of the arena.

Was I scared? I will tell you something now I have never told anyone. For this performance and the eight that followed, I never opened my eyes. Not even a peek. I don't know what that rattler was doing, but I kinda figured that whatever it was, my staring him in the eye was of no benefit to either of us.

I got out of the straitjacket in a minute or so, although I

was careful to make as few unnecessary movements as possible. The jacket off, I reached out with my hands, untied the bag from around my neck, and held it beneath me as the cable lowered me to the ground.

I'd suggest you read the last five or six paragraphs eight more times to get some idea of what I went through that week. I couldn't help feeling that my luck would run out and the snake might eventually take a nip off the top of my head.

The truth is (divulged for the first time) that Battson and I had put a few safeguards in place. First, the snake was iced down half an hour before each performance, which put him in a more tranquil state—still potentially lethal, but less apt to strike. In addition, Battson suggested that the snake spend a few nights before the circus sleeping with my underwear—underwear that we had soaked in my urine, sweat, spit, and hair.

The theory here was that when my head came into the bag, we'd be old friends already. Another questionable theory, but any comfort zone did make me feel better.

In addition, Battson assured me that it was difficult for a snake to bite someone on the top of the head. The angle is wrong; it's hard to bite a round surface; a head is hard; the hair is also a partial protection. I trusted Battson. But it was the snake I still wasn't sure of.

I did nine performances, 60 feet in the air, in a straitjacket with my head in a bag with a rattlesnake. Each one a success. The crowd loved it; they were on the edge of their seats. But I didn't know for sure. Remember, I had my head in a bag with my eyes closed.

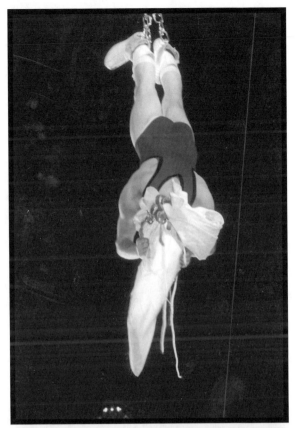

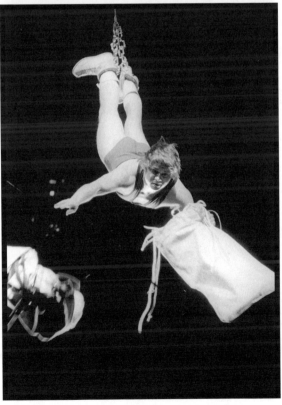

2 Cecil Court, London Road
Enfield, Middlesex EN2 6DJ
Telephone : 01 367 4567
Telegrams and cables : MOSTEST ENFIELD
Telex : 23573

Guinness Superlatives Limited

A MEMBER OF THE GUINNESS GROUP OF COMPANIES

PUBLISHERS

7th July

Mr. William S Poorman
3003 Kessler Blvd.
N Drive
Indianapolis
Indiana
U S A

Dear Mr. Poorman

Just a few lines to acknowledge receipt of your letter of June 26, enclosing the
details and authentication of Bill Shirk's Escape from a regulation straitjacket
whilst suspended below a helicopter, at an altitude of 200'.

This is in orde4r and has been accepted for inclusion in the forthcoming (17th
edition) of the Guinness Book of World Records. This means that Bill will hold
all four world records in Escapology.

The new edition will, we hope, be published as usual in October this year and if
you think that you will require a number of the books at that time, it might be
a good idea for you to approach our United States publishers on the matter ahead
of this date. For your ready reference, the address is:-

Sterling Publishing Co. Inc.,
2 Park Avenue
New York
N Y 10016
U S A

Telephone No. 212-532-7160

You will probably know that the Sterling Publishing Co. run the "Guinness Hall
of World Records" situated in the Empire State Building in New York and it
would not do any harm if you did have a contract with Sterling from the publicity
and show business angle.

With kind regards,

Yours sincerely

G. HOWARD GARRARD
Correspondence Editor
Guinness Book of Records.

P.S. The name of Sterling's president
is DAVID A. BOEHM

Record Performance

FOLLOWING MY SHRINE CIRCUS APPEARANCE,
I was pretty certain that I would retain the four world records
in the 1979 edition of the *Guinness Book*, but I eagerly, almost
obsessively, waited for a letter from the publishers confirming
this. If I wasn't in the book, I wasn't number one. It didn't
matter how many press clippings or how much video I had. I
needed to be in the *Guinness Book of World Records*. Four
times, at least.

The letter finally came and with it some more good news.
The publishers were passing my name along to producer
David Frost for possible inclusion in his Guinness TV show
the coming spring. Frost owned the TV rights to any telecast of
Guinness record holders wanting to promote their talent or
trying to break their own records. I was pumped.

And more good news. The Guinness people were going to
feature me in two of their other publications: the *Guinness
Book of Amazing People* and the *Guinness Book of Daring
Deeds*.

Then even more good news. Calls from Mike Douglas
and Bob Braun for their syndicated TV talk shows. Everything
seemed to be going my way.

Except money. If money was going my way, it just kept
passing me by. And now I needed it more than ever. My AM
radio station had taken a hit by the encroachment of FM. For
the first time we were spending more than we were making.

It was slowly becoming apparent that daredevil stunts were
not big moneymakers. TV shows paid pretty much what they
call "scale," which in circus talk is peanuts. Other venues did
not necessarily have the funds to pay me and, quite frankly,
places like the Shrine Circus felt they were doing me a favor
by giving me an opportunity to market my talent. There was
actually some truth in that.

Truth, but no money.

I was not going to let that get me down, at least not at this

> The letter finally came
> and with it some more
> good news. The
> publishers were
> passing my name along
> to producer David Frost
> for possible inclusion
> in his Guinness TV
> show the coming
> spring.

time. I was going to Hollywood to be on national TV. The money would follow. Wouldn't it?

I arrived in Hollywood to tape the Guinness show. If ever there was a *Who's Who* of people who had chosen bizarre activities to fill their lives, this was the group. Of course, I was in no position to pass judgment, having spent a week with my head in a bag with a rattlesnake. But these people really were strange.

Let me introduce a few folks I got close to and one guy I was afraid to get too close to: That would be Don Cook, the guy with a beard consisting of one queen bee and 17,500 of her slaves and suitors—Italian honeybees covered him from his chin to his waist.

Also:

A man who blew up hot water bottles until they burst.

A man who walked on 25-foot stilts.

A man who with his teeth held back a helicopter from taking off.

A man who had walked on a 2-inch-diameter cable to the top of a mountain in Rio de Janeiro—the very same cable that carried the cable cars to the 2,400-foot summit.

A man who dived 40 feet from a platform into 121/2 inches of water.

All world-record holders. All nice people. And all certifiably nuts. But all smart enough to know that none of them was getting rich with this world-record stuff. And they all tried to impress upon me that if I thought this was my ticket to the good life, I was making a mistake.

Still, I couldn't think about money right now. The first order of business was my performance for the TV show. The potential crowd for this telecast was huge, in the millions, an opportunity I did not want to blow.

I began by lobbying the producers for the best TV time slot for my record-breaking attempt. I wanted to bridge the gap between the two halves of the hour-long show, which meant that the beginning of my escape would start just before the half-hour break and would continue after the commercial.

Specifically, I opted for breaking the world record for getting out of a straitjacket while hanging from a helicopter

Let me introduce a few folks I got close to and one guy I was afraid to get too close to: That would be Don Cook, the guy with a beard consisting of one queen bee and 17,500 of her slaves and suitors— Italian honeybees covered him from his chin to his waist.

200 feet in the air. I would be upside down and attached to the cable by a pair of ice skates. My record of 18.83 seconds, which was in the 1979 *Guinness Book*, had already been broken by Jimmy Dixon of Las Vegas. While I would still hold the title for the 1979 edition, I was already looking ahead to 1980 where he would now trump me unless I could surpass his new record time of 14.9 seconds.

I knew that all eyes would *not* be exclusively on me. I wasn't used to that. I had always craved and sought being the center of attention, so sharing that limelight was a little disconcerting and deflating to the ego. I was in a crowd of performers whose very existence screamed, *Hey, look at me!*, so I knew that my escape had to be stellar. Stand by for what I did.

Once again we had problems getting a helicopter. There was still reluctance by the FAA to allow us to carry a live external load. It was frustrating. You would think Guinness would have some pull in a situation like this. How can a guy find a million bees for his beard and I can't find one helicopter? If you ever want to get into Guinness, blow up hot-water bottles. They're everywhere.

But Guinness did find a chopper. The show began. I was placed in a straitjacket. But, as you'll see, I had something up my sleeve—actually more like in my shoe—that surprised even the Guinness people. The helicopter lifted me to a height of 200 feet. I could be clearly seen by the audience below as I hung below the chopper from a cable attached to my two ice skates. I was told that Gavin MacLeod, the celebrity emcee and host of the Guinness show, was transfixed watching me from his broadcast booth. To ensure the best view for the crowd, I had dyed the straitjacket a chocolate brown so it would contrast with the sky.

The official time commenced when I released a flag from my mouth. The flag dropped—and then so did everyone's jaw as I kicked off the left skate. My free foot actually came down and whacked me on the head. It appeared to the crowd that this was unintentional and that ultimately I would come out of the other skate as well. I couldn't hear the gasps, but I had developed a pretty good sense of when something worked perfectly. This was a winner.

I knew that all eyes would not be exclusively on me. I wasn't used to that. I had always craved and sought being the center of attention, so sharing that limelight was a little disconcerting and deflating to the ego.

I started counting down. I had no exact way to know the time, but ideally I wanted to break Jimmy Dixon's record and still leave a little room for me to break my own in the future. Fourteen, thirteen, twelve, eleven, ten, nine, eight, seven, six, five, four, three, two, one. As I reached what I thought was the fourteenth second, I popped off the jacket, kicked it clear, and watched it spiral to the ground 200 feet below. Total time: 14.7 seconds. Another world record. And on national television!

The decision to release my foot from the skate provided me with two advantages. It significantly increased the PR value of the escape, giving people a little something extra to talk about. Even MacLeod, the emcee, was visibly shaken, I was later told. And several of my quirky associates said they were concerned for me. Don Cook, my bee-bearded friend, said a few prayers for me. With his gig, I figured he did a lot of praying.

Once my left foot was free of the skate, I could use it to help push off the straitjacket, a technique I had learned from Tom Ewing in my pursuit of the land straitjacket record. Fortunately, that technique worked quite well in the air, also.

The event was a success. The escape aired on TV a month later and was seen by thirty-one million people. Keep this in mind: Thirty-one million people is more people than Harry Houdini performed in front of in his whole life. I love to make that point, but it still wasn't money in the bank.

Yes, I might have been more famous then, but I was certainly no richer than I had been before I took my life in my hands. My Guinness colleagues had done a pretty good job of dousing my optimism when it came to future financial security.

Yes, I might have been more famous then, but I was certainly no richer than I had been before I took my life in my hands. My Guinness colleagues had done a pretty good job of dousing my optimism when it came to future financial security.

One thing kept me going. I knew that Harry Houdini had been the highest-paid performer of his time. He had somehow found a way to turn his amazing skills into cash. What was I missing? The answer, I thought, was an agent. Someone who not only recognized my unique skills, but also knew how to utilize my talents in a financially beneficial way. Let me translate that: I needed work. And I needed to save my radio station.

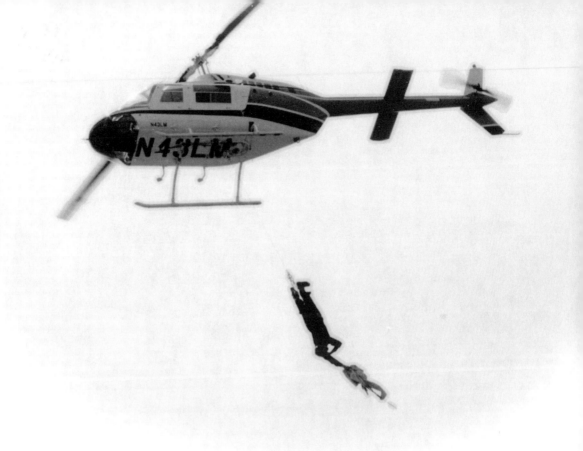

It was then that the Guinness people told me that my old nemesis, Jimmy Dixon, had retaken the ground straitjacket record with a time of 2.4 seconds. That meant that in less than two years, the record had gone from twenty-four seconds to less than three.

I wasn't going to take that sitting down. In fact, I was going to take it standing up.

When I got back to Indy, I paid a visit to the Marion County Sheriff's Training Center. There, with the assistance of Deputy Dave Lewis and in front of twenty other deputies and a video camera, I established a new world record of 1.68 seconds.

That record still stands today, although it is not listed in the current editions of the *Guinness Book* because in 1986 Guinness dropped the "Escapology" category, concerned that people might endanger their lives trying to break these records. If you call Guinness today and ask who has the standing straitjacket record, they'll tell you Bill Shirk. But ya gotta call. You can't look it up.

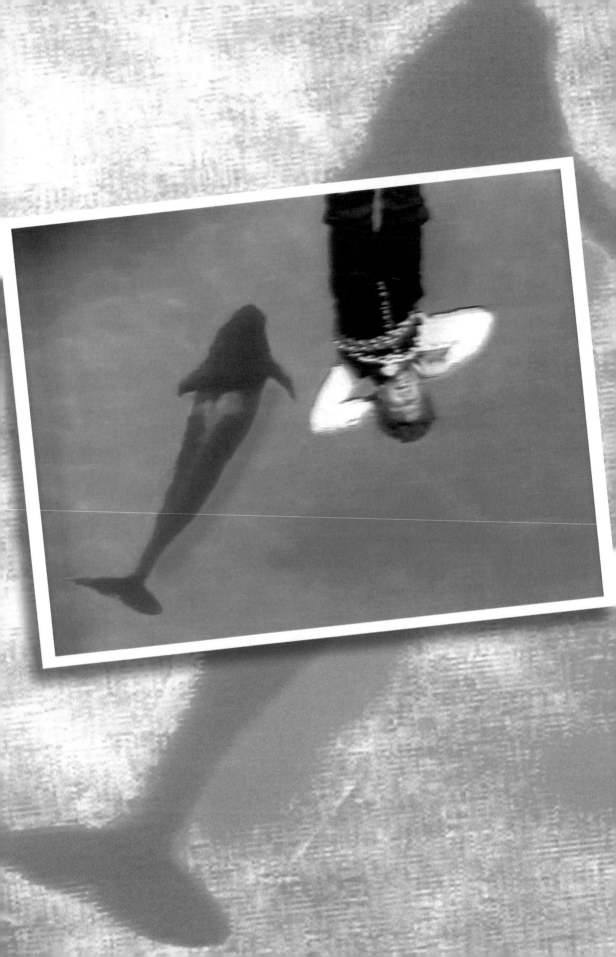

Whale of an Escape

YES, IT WAS TIME FOR AN AGENT. My AM radio station had been in the red, eaten alive by the power of all the new FM stations. I needed to make a total format change. I even considered giving my station to God, switching to an all-religious format. I needed to make money fast. Actually, at that point I just needed to save money fast.

It would be nice to say that I wasn't doing all this for the money, but that would be a lie. While it was true that I did enjoy the adulation from the crowd, there was nothing about my daredevil activities that brought me any pleasure.

I was envious of sports figures, actors, even TV anchors, who not only made a good living but also looked forward to practicing their craft. Sorry to disillusion you, but no one in his right mind looks forward to spending time in a coffin with a rattlesnake or dangling from a burning rope. In fact, despite all the jokes to the contrary, that's how I knew I was in my right mind. I didn't enjoy the escapes. If I had actually enjoyed them, well, then I deserved to be hauled away in a straitjacket—which would have lasted about 1.68 seconds.

Having an agent was not an idea that just popped into my head overnight. I had been sending press clippings to the International Management Group for two years, giving them a sense of who I was, knowing full well that I would, at some point, make an official request for representation.

I finally contacted Mark McCormick of IMG. I was starting at the top. McCormick represented Arnold Palmer, Jack Nicklaus, and Björn Borg. If someone was number one in his field, McCormick represented him. I was Number One. Was there any chance he'd take me on as a client? I honestly didn't think so, but I took a chance. I was good at taking chances.

My letter to McCormick was immodest, to say the least. I bragged about everything from running with the bulls to hanging from a helicopter. I compared myself to Houdini,

> Sorry to disillusion you, but no one in his right mind looks forward to spending time in a coffin with a rattlesnake or dangling from a burning rope.

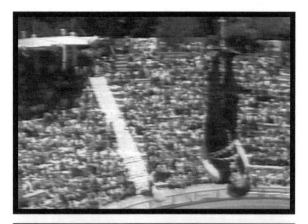

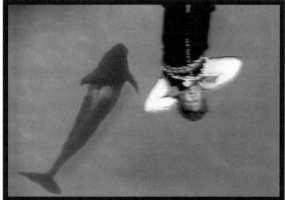

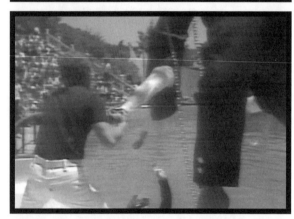

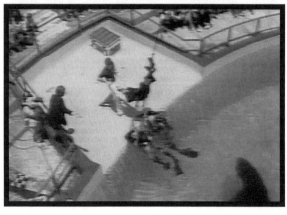

reminding McCormick of the tremendous marketing potential for acts like these.

The bad news is that I wasn't sure I believed half of what I said. The good news is that Mark McCormick did. I was incredulous. I was going to be represented by the same company that represented Muhammad Ali. Was this the ticket to fame and fortune I was waiting for? I thought so.

It wasn't long before McCormick and his number one man, Barry Frank, had a gig for me on *NBC's Sports World*, a popular network show that featured sporting events and athletic-related stunts. It couldn't have been more perfect. They were going to pay me $15,000. That was $15,000 more than anyone had ever paid me before.

And what did they want me to do for fifteen grand? They weren't quite sure, so they asked me to provide three choices — three options that could wow a huge audience in person and on national television. Here's what I suggested:

1. Hang from the Empire State Building in a straitjacket.
2. Hang upside down in a straitjacket with a 14-foot python around me.
3. Hang from a burning rope, while handcuffed and chained, over a pool of thirty sharks.

For each of these escapes, I planned a powerful climax. I promised to crash through a glass window when hanging from the Empire State Building; to be strangled by the python; and finally, if they picked number three, I would allow the rope to burn in two, sending me into the tank of sharks.

They picked number three. I could have guessed. The movie *Jaws* was the current number one box-office attraction. It was perfect timing again.

The original plan was for me to fly to Los Angeles, but a change in scheduling meant that the venue would move to San Francisco. No big deal, right? Wrong! After consulting with my brother, the expert in marine life, I discovered that they were not just changing venues, they were changing sharks. Bob did some research and was pretty clear about what this meant . . .

"Bill, the sharks in L.A. are blue sharks; you have a chance to survive if you get out in a minute or so; they swim with the trainers sometimes; they're sweethearts, like Larry's rattlesnake. In San Francisco, they're bull sharks; not friendly, not predictable. Not a good idea."

There was more. Bob told me that I would be hanging over the feeding tank. The place where the sharks were fed red meat every day. The sharks would consume anything in that tank. And I would eventually be in that tank.

I called Barry Frank and pleaded my case. Boy, did I plead. Frank was understanding. Nothing was more important to him than my safety—next to cutting his traveling expenses, that is.

We needed an alternative. And we found one. Orca the Killer Whale was alive and well and swimming in San Francisco at Marine World. Bob confirmed with the trainers that the huge mammal was basically playful, often toying with her trainers. Unfortunately, the whale's idea of play often involved keeping her toy underwater for a minute or so.

"Okay," I told Barry Frank, "I'll do it. I'll hang from a burning rope handcuffed and chained over the pool. The rope will burn in two and I will fall into the pool with Orca the Killer Whale."

"I like the sound of that," said Frank. "Will you still be alive?"

"Yes."

"We have a deal."

The event was set for Marine World in San Francisco, where we would tape in front of 12,000 people; the show would then be aired on TV in front of millions.

There was more. Bob told me that I would be hanging over the feeding tank. The place where the sharks were fed red meat every day. The sharks would consume anything in that tank. And I would eventually be in that tank.

The night before my scheduled 6:00 A.M. call for setup and preparation, I decided to celebrate my good fortune with some old fraternity brothers who lived in the Bay Area. So here I was, less than twelve hours from the opportunity of a lifetime slamming down brewskies in some San Francisco saloon. Real smart, Bill.

At three in the morning, I left the bar knowing that if I got right home I might be able to squeeze in a couple of hours of sleep. My head was throbbing. What had I done?

As I cut through an alley to the hotel, a friendly neighborhood hoodlum put a knife to my back. I could tell you more about this incident, but this book is not about great robberies, it's about great escapes. I wouldn't call this one an escape; he just let me go. I thanked him by giving him all the cash in my wallet.

The whole evening had become like a bad dream. I staggered back to the hotel. Bob, my brother, was asleep. After all, he had a big day coming up. He was going to watch me kill myself. I stuck my head in the shower. In case you want to know, that never works.

The morning was only hours away. I barely slept, just hoping this was a dream and I would wake up with a clear head. It wasn't and I didn't. I had thought that last night's headache was big, but this was worse. Wait a second, this *was* last night's headache.

Believe it or not, I arrived at Marine World at 6:00 A.M. as scheduled and learned that Lady Orca was in heat. This may not mean a lot to you, but Orca's mate was in a nearby pool, and he thought that this was just about the most important thing going. My brother told me that the whole situation could make Mrs. Orca a little edgy. Great. An edgy killer whale.

It was ninety degrees. I was to wear a solid black suit for the escape. The arena was open at the top, but inside the air circulation was very poor. You couldn't make up a worse set of circumstances. I took a handful of aspirin. I was nauseous. I could see the headlines the next day:

SHIRK HURLS FROM BURNING ROPE

I managed to make my way to the stage where a huge

> **At three in the morning, I left the bar knowing that if I got right home I might be able to squeeze in a couple of hours of sleep. My head was throbbing. What had I done?**

crane was to hoist me upside down and place me over the pool. The local sheriff fitted me with the chains and handcuffs, then lit the rope just a couple of feet above my head. Up, up I went.

Even in my condition, I did manage to successfully unlock the handcuffs with a concealed pick and then release myself from the chains. I was beginning to almost look forward to a dip in the cool water, although I must admit that *killer whale in heat* had an ominous ring to it.

Two minutes had passed. The rope should have burned by now. I looked up. The rope wasn't burning. Moisture from the ocean and the pool had saturated the line and the flame had flickered out. It was only later that I realized I had always done the burning rope escape inside. Outside was a whole different story.

There was nothing I could do. Nothing anyone could do. I did try to bounce on the rope, hoping some added pressure might snap the line, but it had not burned nearly enough. I even reached up to try to break the rope, but it was still very hot and I charred my fingers and palm.

The sun beat down on me. I started to hyperventilate. I was in serious trouble. Then, twenty-two minutes later, I passed out. Dead out. I'm not talking about feeling woozy, or spacey, or groggy. I'm talking flat-out unconscious. Upside down.

The next thing I remembered was waking up in the hospital. My brother had a sensitive question . . .

"Bill, are you faking this?"

"Faking what?" I said. "Where the hell am I?"

No, I wasn't faking. It was all too real. I did get the fifteen grand, but I knew my agent was disappointed with the outcome. After all, I was in charge of the stunt. It didn't work, so who else could he blame? Of course, the segment never aired. A guy passing out upside down on a rope, even in 1979, was not Must-See TV.

Nothing had changed back home. The radio station was in trouble. I was in debt. I felt my recent failed escape would define my career.

If you'll excuse the expression: I was lower than killer whale shit.

The sun beat down on me. I started to hyperventilate. I was in serious trouble. Then, twenty-two minutes later, I passed out. Dead out. I'm not talking about feeling woozy, or spacey, or groggy. I'm talking flat-out unconscious. Upside down.

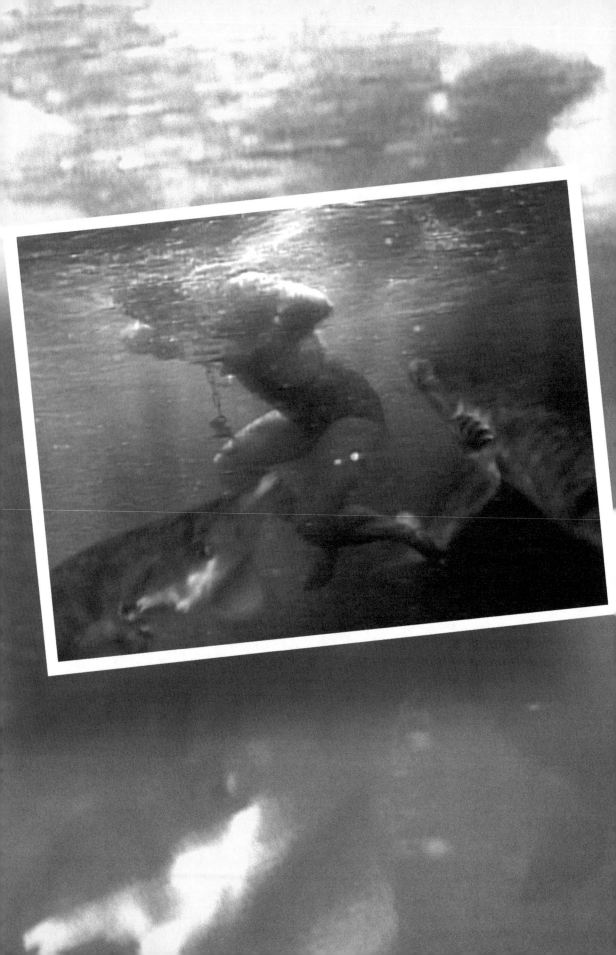

Jaws of Death

I WAS DEVASTATED BY MY LAST ESCAPE attempt, and my radio station was in the dumps. What does a guy like me do when he's depressed?

It was time to be reborn and get religion. In radio talk, thats a format change to all-Christian programming, a move I made to save my hide and conserve money. The change allowed me to cut staff, including jocks and newspeople. I didn't want to do it, but I had no choice.

But by giving up the traditional format, I was also reliquishing my major vehicle for PR. I was like Houdini without his magic show.

Yeah, I was pretty down. Suddenly a miracle: a phone call gave me just the lift I needed. It was International Management Group again. At first I thought they were going to bitch some more about the nonburning rope, but instead they wanted to use that failed attempt as the basis of a new appearance on network TV.

The show was called *Games People Play* on NBC and it was a spin-off of ABC's *That's Incredible*, a program that had been plagued by stunt-makers who had been hurt badly, including one guy who lost his foot and another who caught on fire. I guess they thought I had a pretty good track record at not getting myself dead or hurt too badly. And that it would be neat to play off my recent failure, then do a follow-up to see if I could complete the escape properly. In fact, they wanted me to do the escape as I had originally planned it—not over a whale in heat, but over a tank of sharks.

There was one additional request from IMG. "Bill, the network wants to film you out on a fishing boat actually catching the blue sharks that will be in the tank you'll fall into. That will prove they are wild and vicious."

"Gee, what a great idea!" I said, once again agreeing to something I had not completely thought out. Oh, and by the way, blue sharks were responsible for the most recorded human attacks on the L.A. coast. Did you know that? I didn't either.

> **"Bill, the network wants to film you out on a fishing boat actually catching the blue sharks that will be in the tank you'll fall into. That will prove they are wild and vicious."**

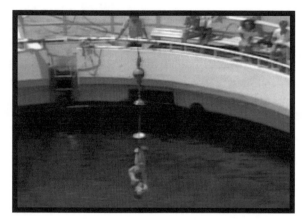

Then I started to think about it. Plunging into a tank with a dozen sharks that had just been involuntarily relocated from their home didn't seem like a very good idea. Especially if I was depending on them to be in relatively good spirits during my surprise visit. This seemed a pretty long way from Larry Battson's assurance, "This rattlesnake is a sweetheart. Not to worry."

I thought about it for three seconds.

"Let's do it," I heard myself say. I might have taken longer to decide, but the offer of another fifteen grand speeded up my thinking considerably.

"And don't screw up the rope burning," they reminded me. "Or you won't get the money."

A couple of weeks later I was on my way to L.A. I arrived at the dock and met Shark Roberts. Yes, that was his name, and he reminded me of Robert Shaw in the movie *Jaws*. And his boat was in no better shape.

Despite the big hype about filming this fishing trip for the

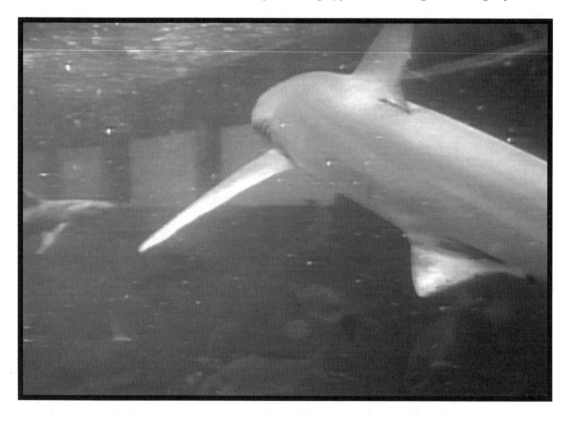

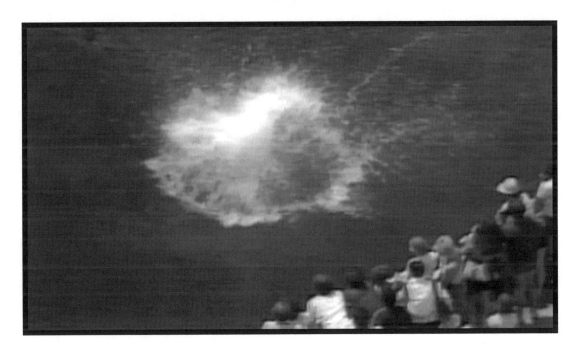

show, the TV crew never showed up, making me question the commitment they had to the entire idea. A still photographer did come to take pictures, but I was disappointed that the production company had not followed through with their original concept.

Roberts's approach to catching these blue sharks was similar to that portrayed in *Jaws*. We went out on the ocean and set out hundreds of yards of fishing cable with dozens of meated hooks, each line connected to a barrel that acted as a huge bobber. Then Roberts chummed the water with fish heads, fish guts, and fish blood, hoping to entice as many blue sharks as possible to take the baited hooks.

It worked. Boy, did it work. We caught more than a dozen blue sharks, all in excess of 5 feet and each one in a bit of a snit about leaving the homeland involuntarily. I knew that the next morning, Bill Shirk the homewrecker would be dropping in unexpectedly to their new digs.

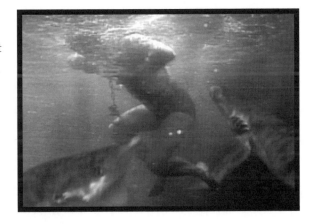

I was having second thoughts.

As nervous as I was about the sharks, I was more concerned with the rope not burning in two. You can die in an escape or your act can die. I was facing both

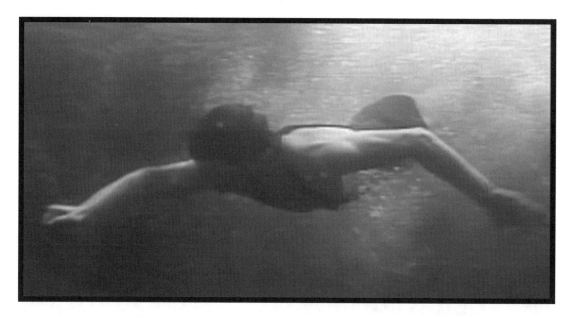

possibilities. I took no chances. I couldn't de-tooth the sharks, but I did ensure the rope would split in two by hooking up a quick-release system. Basically I would control when the rope broke by pulling a wire, rather than depending on the fire, which inevitably burns out before splitting the rope.

The day of the show arrived. I was cuffed and chained, once again by a local sheriff. That was thirty pounds of chain. A nice outfit to wear when you're plunging to the bottom of a huge aquarium. The crane hoisted me up feet first. They lit the rope and the countdown began. I feigned fighting with the restraints, knowing full well that it would be far more dramatic if I plunged into the water completely chained and then escaped.

The pool was surrounded by 2,000 people and a handful of photographers, all of whom could see me through the clear tank at eye level. After two minutes, I released the rope and plummeted 20 feet into the water. Along with the twelve blue sharks, there were twenty other sharks—a total of thirty-two, but only about a dozen of them man-eaters, I was told. I guess that was supposed to make me feel safer.

I hit the water. The thirty pounds of chain dragged me to the bottom. To be honest, I didn't have much time to think about the sharks. I was literally anchored to the bottom and had only a minute or so to get out of the chains before I'd drown. If I did drown, I'd be dead meat. Sharks like dead meat.

They lit the rope and the countdown began. I feigned fighting with the restraints, knowing full well that it would be far more dramatic if I plunged into the water completely chained and then escaped.

I released myself in about forty seconds. The sharks were circling me. They didn't seem very happy, although I'm not sure what a happy shark looks like. Moments later I reached the side of the pool and scrambled out. I did have a vision of losing a foot in the final moments, but the escape was clean. And the crowd loved it.

I haven't told you the whole story. This was a dangerous escape, but not nearly as risky as the audience (and you) thought. I had an edge no one knew about. But you will, now.

True, the blue sharks were dangerous in their natural habitat, but my marine biologist brother had assured me of two things: First, the sharks would be in a state of partial shock from being moved from the ocean. And in cases like this, they would not feed for several days. Second, sharks usually circle before attacking their prey, and my plan was to get out quick. Real quick.

And what about those handcuffs and chains? No, I didn't use a pick or key. Houdini knew that a water escape did not have a margin of error. If the pick was hard to reach or fell out of my hand, I was shark chow, anchored to the bottom of the tank, running out of air. I'd be a sitting duck. Sharks like duck, also. Even dead ducks.

No, I had a different plan of escape. In a daring sleight of hand, I switched the handcuffs they were going to use with an identical set that I had shaved the day before. Shaved handcuffs are easy to pull out of because the sawteeth inside have been leveled, preventing them from catching when the cuffs are closed. A good hard tug and I would be free.

A successful escape. National attention and exposure followed over the next few weeks, including a caricature in *TV Guide*. The radio station was starting to do better, and I started living with Liz, a girlfriend who would one day be my wife.

I have admitted to you that doing these escapes was not something I looked forward to.

Imagine how Liz felt.

If the pick was hard to reach or fell out of my hand, I was shark chow, anchored to the bottom of the tank, running out of air. I'd be a sitting duck. Sharks like duck, also. Even dead ducks.

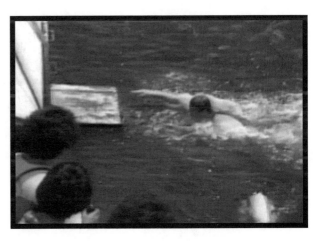

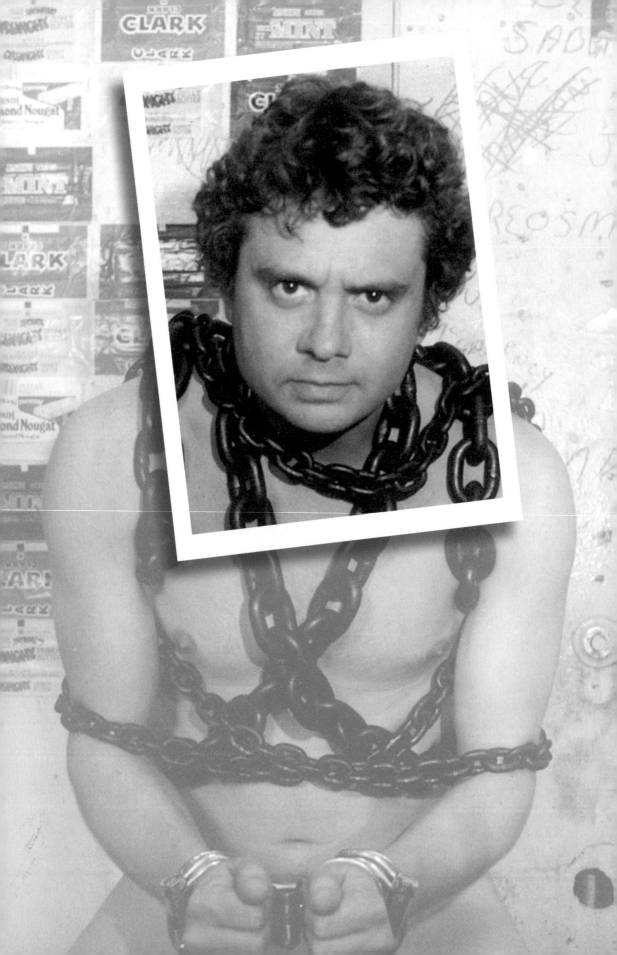

Movie Madness

THE EARLY 1980'S WERE A LOW POINT FOR ME. My beloved father passed away and I found myself dealing with intense grief while still trying to juggle some serious business setbacks. Then I discovered that two of my escape records in the 1981 *Guinness Book* had been eliminated as a category for future printings. All that remained was the 1.68-second straitjacket escape and the jail escape. Even *that* would be eliminated in 1986.

So what do you do when your life seems like a bad movie? You make a movie about your life. And guess what?—and I should have predicted this—it turned out to be a bad movie, too.

The first rumblings of this ill-fated idea began in 1982 when I began entertaining the notion that a movie

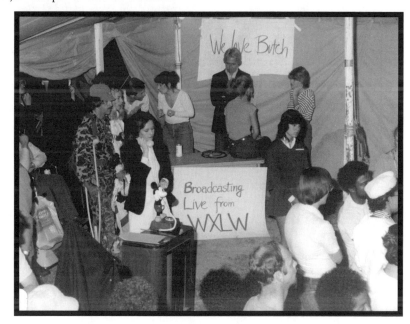

about me would help preserve my legacy—and get several of the escapes down on film as well.

I collaborated with an old college buddy, Steve Meyers, who was a screenwriter, and then teamed up with director Eddie Beverly, who had worked on a few low-budget movies. We managed to find thirty-three investors at ten grand apiece, raising more than $300,000 for the project.

The very idea of making a movie in Indiana was unique. Oh, there were a slew of movies *about* Indiana, but actually filming in the Hoosier State was rare. In fact, we couldn't find a record of a single motion picture completely shot and produced in Indiana. This was one of only two states that didn't even have a film commission.

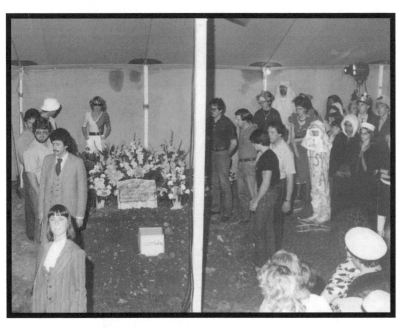

When word leaked of my plans, in part due to an *Indianapolis News* column by David Mannweiller, the response was overwhelmingly positive. Even then-Mayor Hudnut and Lieutenant Governor Mutz were on the bandwagon, hoping this would be the beginning of a trend to make Indy the next Hollywood. Yeah, right!

I was smart enough to hire a film crew from L.A., but the majority of actors and actresses were my friends.

This was all very heady, even for a guy used to a fair amount of adulation. Here I was, making a film about my life, the story of a small-time AM radio station owner plagued with financial problems who goes to Hollywood to make it big. Yes, this was a story about exactly what I was doing. People told me this was a brilliant idea. These same people also wanted parts in the movie.

I didn't really know what I was getting into. Selling an independent film requires considerable business savvy, but I lacked experience in this very specialized area, and that proved to be financially fatal.

I was smart enough to hire a film crew from L.A., but the majority of actors and actresses were my friends. (At least they were when the movie began.) The terms *actors* and *actresses* are probably a bit of an exaggeration. The exceptions were Dick the Bruiser, a natural actor, and Milbourne Christopher who turned a stellar performance his first and only time appearing in a movie. I also asked almost every local radio personality to be in the cast, assuming they would promote the movie when it was released.

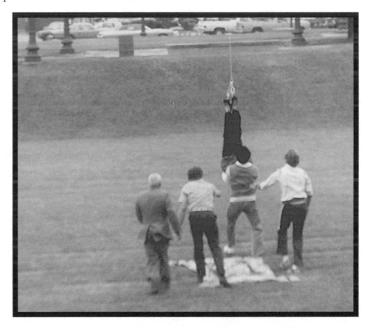

There is something about being in a movie that has an almost diabolical effect on human beings. People would say: "Shirk, I'll die if I'm not in that movie." Of course, many almost died just by virtue of their performances. I barely survived myself.

Later, we'll talk about Shirk, the actor. On second thought, maybe we won't. First, I was Shirk the executive producer—a man with a huge ego was now in charge of scores of people who also now had huge egos. But I was old ego. Many of these people were getting a huge ego for the first time and they didn't know how to handle it. It was dangerous.

Speaking of dangerous, I had to make some important decisions about the stunts I was to perform. In theory this was just a movie; I did not have quite the same obligation to do things for real as I would in a live escape. But I saw the movie as a chance to capture some of my stunts on film, and I also knew that any talk of these scenes being rigged or faked would be detrimental to my reputation. Guinness may not have recognized all my records, but that didn't mean I didn't still hold them.

I decided to re-create six escapes for the film. The first was the helicopter escape, this time from 1,800 feet, hanging from one skate in 25-mile-per-hour winds. I was also buried alive, now accompanied by a 10-foot python, two tarantulas, and—ready for this?—a cobra. For the movie, an extensive time underground was not necessary, but as you will see later in this chapter, I would ultimately spend more time underground for this movie than for any escape or stunt before.

I was also buried alive, now accompanied by a 10-foot python, two tarantulas, and—ready for this?—a cobra.

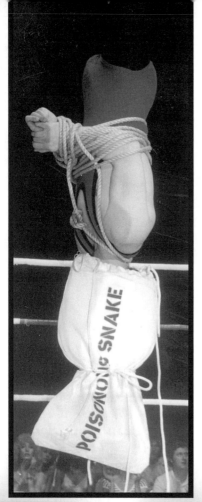

The third escape was performed at the Shrine Circus, a re-creation of the burning rope stunt, where I hung from the ceiling in a straitjacket with a 14-foot python draped around me.

A fourth escape was back to the head-in-the-bag with a rattlesnake. In this case, I did substitute a friendlier reptile, but that proved not to eliminate the real danger: The quick release on the rope that held me upside down malfunctioned, and I fell 18 feet onto my back. While the X-rays were inconclusive, I would learn years later that I had actually cracked three ribs. So intense was the pain that I had begged my doctor for a narcotic painkiller, despite his warnings of some unpredictable side effects. I popped those pills for several days while I performed the helicopter escape in 9.8 seconds and broke my own world record of 14.7 seconds. The doctor was right, however: For almost three years, I could not taste or smell anything.

The fifth stunt may sound very tantalizing in print, but I am here to warn you not to try it at home. Or at the office, for that matter. Part of the movie's story involved my relationship with a stripper. Following one of my escapes, we returned to my apartment for a bit of romance. In the bedroom scene, you see my lady friend and me both suspended from the ceiling making love upside down, hanging from our heels. This

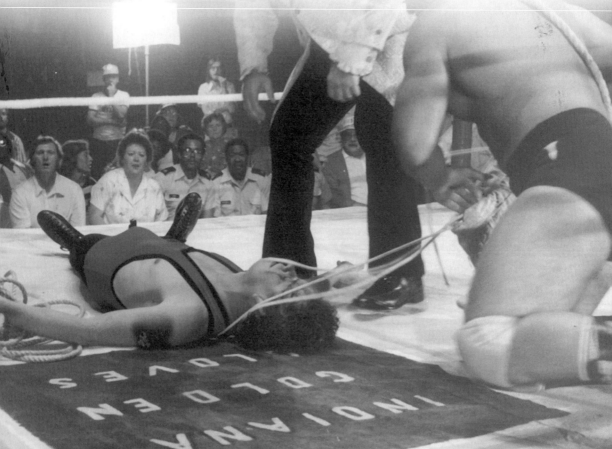

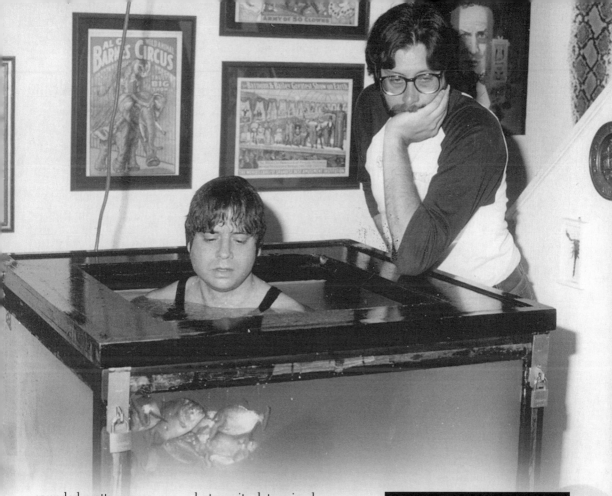

sounded pretty sexy on paper, but gravity determined
movement of body parts and muscles during our embrace—
which made me realize why apes come out of the trees for sex.
I know this fantasy-rich scenario sounds very inviting, but I can
tell you that when you are upside down with cameras on you
and people are watching, it is difficult for a man to get it down.
That's a bad joke, but it's the only thing in this whole chapter
that's really given me a smile so far.

Within weeks of production, I realized that we were in a
financial mess. Costs sneak up on you from every direction,
costs you would not anticipate unless you had experience
making a movie: meals, insurance, site fees, costumes,
makeup. I saw what little money we had quickly begin to
dwindle.

Debt increased, egos got larger. Everything got bigger but
the acting talent. At one point many of the crew members
threatened to quit, wanting to distance themselves from me
because they were convinced I was going to kill myself. I was

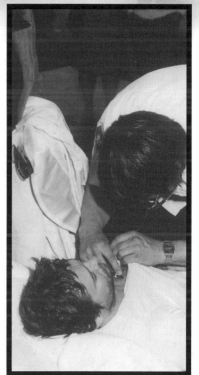

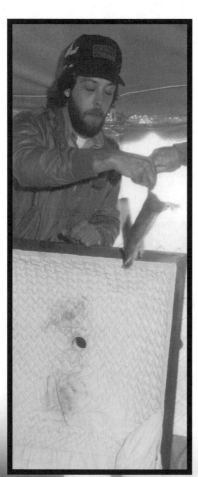

thinking about it, but it would have been a more traditional suicide.

In May 1983 we finished the film, one year after we began shooting. At this point I was in debt to the tune of $180,000 and I had hocked my radio station so that we could complete the film and start making some serious money.

I even hit my mom up for sixty grand, tugging at her heartstrings by reminding her that the movie was dedicated to my late father. Mom was not a big fan of my escapes, but she knew how important the movie was to me. She may have been the only person in my life wanting me to finish the movie who wasn't in it. Now that's love.

The world premiere was a huge success. We filled the Eastwood Theater, seating almost 1,000 people. This was 1,000 paying customers, but I had decided to give all the proceeds to charity. A nice gesture, but I did forget that I was in a lot of financial trouble myself.

The sellout crowd gave me a real high. That theater had only been sold out once before, the night of the *Star Wars* opening. This time it was for the first movie shot, financed and produced right here in Indiana. My movie.

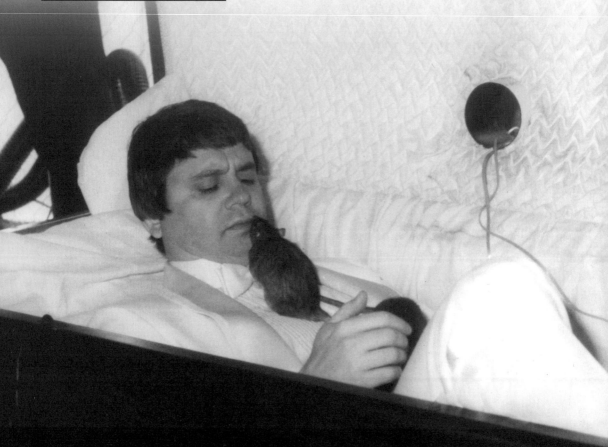

My Son, the Escape Artist

By Betty Poorman

I really don't know why a normal little boy who loved basketball and baseball grew up and decided to put his head in a bag with a rattlesnake, or hang from a rope with a python around his neck. People ask me why all the time. Heavens, I hope it wasn't anything I did.

He was a pretty typical kid who liked helping others. He used to come home from school without his coat, his gloves, or his hat. He was giving them to poor children who didn't have warm clothes. Of course, that was my influence.

The bizarre activities started when he moved down to Indy from Muncie in 1972. Just when he was finally old enough to know better is when he started doing all this crazy stuff.

I've witnessed a few of his stunts but for the most part I can't bear to watch. I saw one burial and that was enough. I'm claustrophobic myself.

I did see him hang from a burning rope. I saw on video the one where the coffin collapses but I'll never watch it again. They call him Crazy Bill. I can't blame them. Just thinking about some of the things he's done gives me goose bumps.

Then there was that movie he made. Not the worst movie ever. Okay, not the best, either. The film is kinda like the burial. Seeing it once is enough.

I gave Bill my last $60,000 in the world so he could finish the film back in 1982. I knew how much that meant to him. He's paid me back many times over.

I hope he's done with all this escape stuff, but I doubt it. You can't predict what Bill will do next. I don't think he knows, either. To be honest, whatever it is, I can't say I'm looking forward to it.

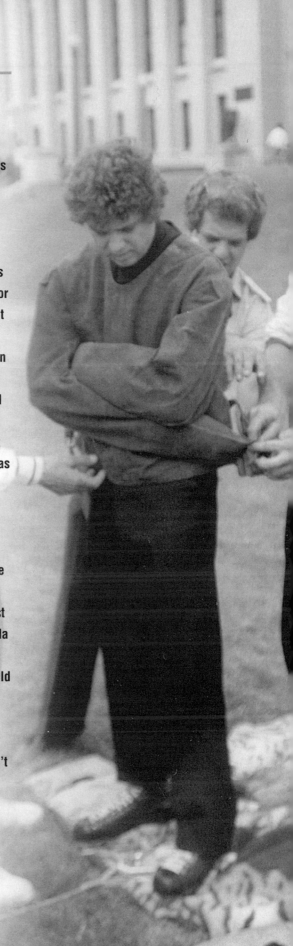

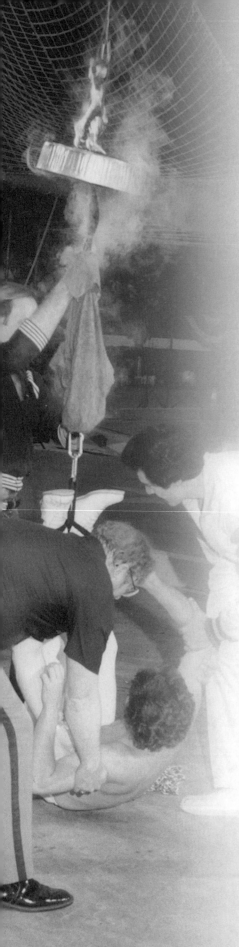

Everyone loved the movie. (Why not? They were all in it.) I saw this as further proof that we were on our way to a huge success. I was so convinced of our future payload that I staged what remains the stupidest publicity stunt of all time.

I pledged to stay underground in a new coffin with half a dozen rats until the Eastwood Theater sold out to a paying audience. This brilliant notion had not taken into account several factors that extended my underground vacation far longer than I had anticipated.

First, despite some good press about the filming of the movie, the media still saw me and my radio station as competition, which meant that once the movie opened, they were not going to give me any free publicity. My own radio station, WXLW, was a small, AM, all-religion channel, and it was unseemly to advertise my activities on the airways.

So there I lay. One day, two days . . . two weeks. Yes, two weeks. Two weeks in a coffin with not a friggin' thing to do but wait until that theater sold out. Even the rats got bored and started attacking each other—not a good sign, because it meant that at some point I would be next. Ultimately I did release the rats through the air tube. Remember, I'm crazy, not stupid.

The theater never sold out. Everyone begged me to come up, but I refused. The burial might have had some promotional value, but then a column by a *Star* critic lambasted the movie. Here I was, underground, and the critics were burying me again.

I needed to save face, assuming I had much of a face left after going without food for two weeks and losing twenty pounds. I said I would come out if Johnny Carson would have me on his show. Carson, whose father had died that week, likely never even got the message; even if he had, he probably would have felt that if he capitulated to my demand, others would have tried similar ploys. And his father was in a grave himself. And he wasn't coming up. Bad timing.

After two weeks it was time to give up. And come up. But I even resisted then. Almost like a prisoner of war, I had grown accustomed to my surroundings. In some ways I felt safe down there. Free from debt, bad movie reviews, and rotten actors. But up I came.

I wasn't the same Bill Shirk. I was paranoid, uncommunicative, and so weak I couldn't even eat. I went home. It was the sorriest day of my life.

It took several weeks to recuperate, physically and emotionally. I was starting to feel better so I headed for Hollywood, trying unsuccessfully to hawk the movie. Door after door was slammed in my face. I did sell the movie to the foreign market for worldwide videotape distribution and managed to recoup some of the money, but overall the entire venture was financially devastating.

At the end of the movie, I'm locked by the villain in a water torture chamber—a huge, glass, water-filled enclosure. The scene shifts to several minutes later when my friends race to my rescue, only to discover my skeletal remains in the tank with a dozen piranhas looking quite content after dining on my flesh.

The camera pans and I am sitting on a nearby couch eating popcorn as though I'm watching a bad movie . . . which I was. Unfortunately, it was mine.

Yeah, my whole life was a bad movie, but Liz became sort of my professional compass. "What you are good at is running radio stations. Concentrate on that and we'll be fine." The woman made sense. So I married her. And I married her on Halloween. I didn't want to end my streak of doing crazy things on October 31.

I could escape anything but my wife's logic. For the next several years, I put most of my energy into building my radio empire. I was a long way from making it big, but my new focus would pay off.

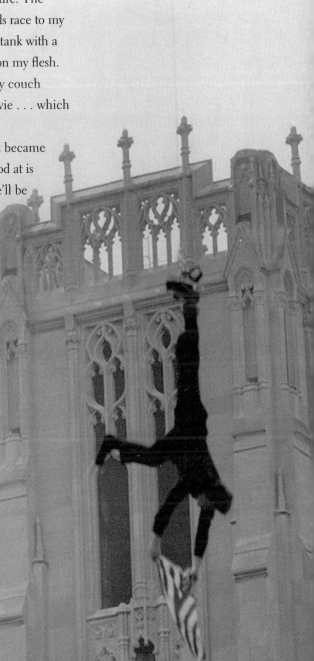

I did not, however, completely give up escapes. I felt a commitment to the Houdini legend and vowed to do an escape each Halloween. But I rethought my motives. I was no longer obsessed with world records or being compensated for my stunts. I tried to look at them as yearly diversions, not life-or-death moments in my career. Of course, some of them could have been life-or-death moments.

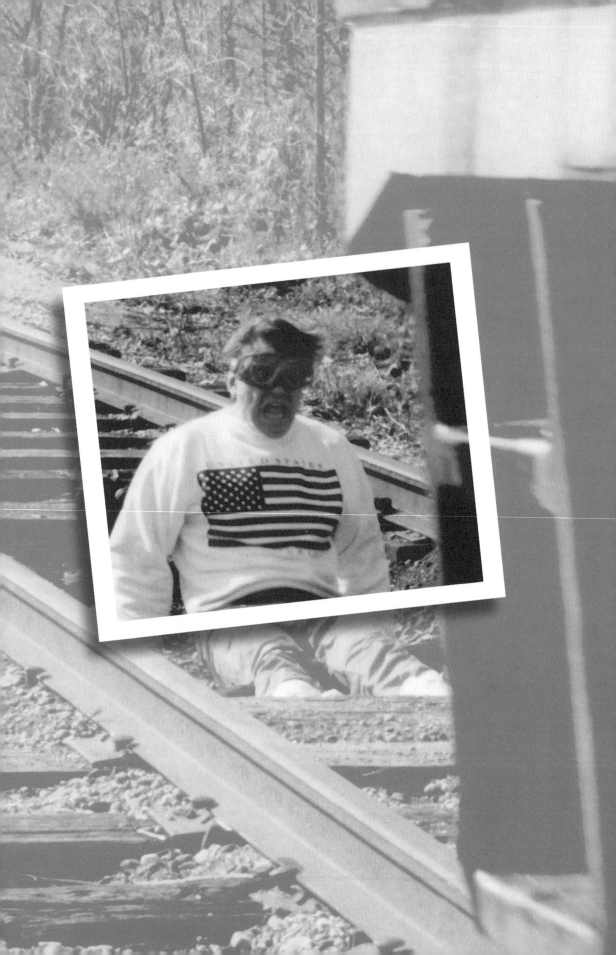

Back on Track

MAGIC IS ALL ILLUSION. But an escape is sometimes a curious combination of illusion and reality. An escape artist who says he spent forty-eight hours underground in a coffin, only to admit he tunneled over to a Holiday Inn for two glorious nights, would lose favor with his fans. It would strike you as fraudulent. You'd feel cheated. You tend to think that you could have done that yourself.

When I exited the coffin after seventy-nine hours back in 1977, I had a snake wrapped around my neck. The illusion was that it had been strangling me for three days. As I have revealed in this book, the snake was really safely tied up in my pants. I removed him in the last few minutes and put him around my throat.

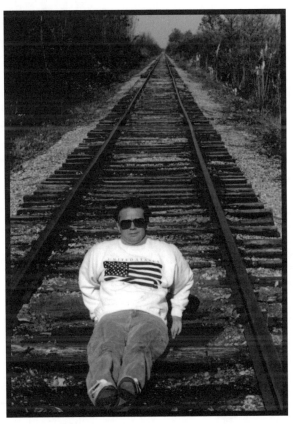

I believe that this illusion is acceptable, because you can then applaud my ingenuity, rather than be put off by the deception. Nevertheless, I created the illusion in order to heighten the effect. But I *was* in the coffin. And it was a *real* python.

In my next escape I was honestly torn between creating a dramatic illusion for the spectator and actually doing something that many were calling suicidal. Here's the story:

It was early in 1990. WXLW had become a successful religious station—maybe the most successful in the state. In addition, I was on the verge of getting a new FM license, thus giving me back my platform to promote my escapes.

To celebrate the anniversary of Houdini's death (again!), I was looking for an escape that was truly unusual. At the time I had written a movie script in which I featured myself as a daredevil motorcyclist who flirts with a speeding train and barely escapes being crushed as he crosses the tracks. The image intrigued me. I researched the history of escapes and could not find any record of any stunt involving facing down a train.

Wouldn't it be exciting to stand on the tracks as a train barreled down on you? Then at the last moment you would fall completely flat between the tracks as the train rolled over you. Playing chicken with a train! Don't you just love it?

But could it be done? Could I find a train? Was there room under the train? I didn't know. And I honestly wasn't sure if I really wanted to perform this stunt or simply create the illusion that I had.

I called David Mannweiller, a fan of my exploits. He published a column about my idea, garnering a very negative response from at least one railroad company that thought the plan was suicidal—and bad publicity for them, to boot. They even cited a Russian psychic who had tried to stop a train with his mental powers and was crushed and splattered all over the Soviet Union. This was not my plan. Once again, *crazy* and *stupid* are two different things.

Ironically, the negative response from this train company, Norfolk & Southern, generated enough PR to sort of beat the bushes for someone willing to help me out. After all, I needed a train. Enter Tom Allison, a good ol' boy who loved my religious station and my escapes, a combination that could not have been better. Or stranger. And he owned his own train. And tracks. And an engineer's hat. What a find!

By the time I met with Allison, I had decided that this was a stunt I needed to do with smoke and mirrors, not guts and brawn. I explained to Allison that I was going to create the illusion of being run over by manipulating the angle at which people watched the stunt, but I needed his help. "It's Halloween," I told him, "let's give 'em a show." He loved it. He was more pumped than me.

I knew one thing. At some point we needed to show the public that this stunt could be done; that there was room for the train to pass over me. This would stem any skepticism and add to the authenticity of the event.

Allison understood what I wanted, but informed me that this pesky nose of mine and my shoes would extend too high

Wouldn't it be exciting to stand on the tracks as a train barreled down on you? Then at the last moment you would fall completely flat between the tracks as the train rolled over you. Playing chicken with a train! Don't you just love it?

up and would be mangled by the locomotive. There just wasn't enough clearance.

Allison didn't want to lose the gig, so he suggested that we cut away three of the railroad ties and dig a kind of cavity in the track which would allow me to rest comfortably as the train screeched over me 3 inches above my nose. Again, this was just for demonstration purposes. I wasn't planning on actually doing this. Was I?

Once this was accomplished, Allison and I began a practice regimen where I stood next to the track, he would barrel down the rails, and I would time my decision to fall back so it appeared that I had successfully avoided the train. The better I timed this, the better it would look. The audience needed to think I had fallen beneath the train and that it would clear my body.

This was not as easy as you might think. I was troubled by my feet kicking up when I hit the track, but repeated practice using my hand during the fall to cushion my butt and reduce the bounce seemed to make a difference.

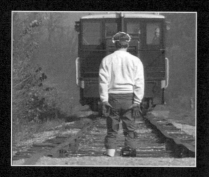

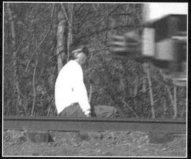

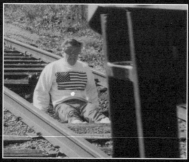

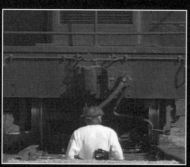

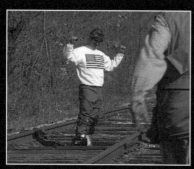

In essence, I was creating an optical illusion. To spectators, it would appear I was standing in the middle of the track when I was actually one foot outside of and adjacent to the track. If I timed it correctly, it would look like the train had come within inches of my nose. Then seconds later I would jump to my feet, again appearing as though I was in the center of the track.

The Norfolk & Southern Railroad actually pursued stopping me legally. In a note to the prosecutor, the railroad brass said: ". . . the stunt would surely result in death or serious injury and I urge you to ask the sheriff and prosecuting attorneys to take steps to prevent it. Don't statues on pre-meditated murder, manslaughter and trespassing apply in this situation?"

The day of the event, Allison and I staged the practice run where I established that I could fit under the train. I lay on the track and Allison very slowly ran over me. Engine oil dripped all over my face. The media was present, including photographers from a European newspaper. They all anxiously awaited the real thing. Not that there was going to be a real thing. It was going to be an illusion. Wasn't it?

We were ready to go. Allison got the train up to full throttle. I stood in the center of the track and walked forward. Then I stepped off to the side of the track. Right on cue, just as we had practiced, I leaned back and flattened myself on the ground as the train came within inches of running me over—or appearing to run me over. To heighten the effect, when the train passed me, I donned a mask; when I popped back up I was all ready for Halloween.

I don't think anyone knew what I really did. I don't think anyone cared. It was almost too easy. Even Mann-weiller, whom I swear saw through this, wrote the story as if I'd actually done it. He accepted the illusion as he would a good magic trick. He didn't question my honesty; he just applauded the effect.

I almost felt guilty.

But it wasn't that simple. I already knew that the

European photographers felt restrained by the angles they were relegated to, and my own production company was frustrated by the shots they had missed. "We really need to get a better view of this," they all said. "Can you do it again?"

So there it was. I'd fooled 'em, but they needed more. And that's when I realized that I might have to *really* do this. Do this thing that people had called suicide. Do it because this may have crossed the line between illusion and outright deception. I had crossed that line on April Fools' Day during the White River swim, but I didn't want to cross it on the anniversary of Houdini's final disappearance.

Yeah, I knew I had to do it for real. Even Liz knew I would never be happy unless I did. *Okay, let's do it*, I said to myself. *Let's do it for real.* Good-bye Liz! She couldn't watch.

We set it all up again. I told Allison we were going to do the exact same thing for the crowd. I hated to lie to him, but I feared he'd refuse.

The train backed up. I got back on the track. The train started to chug and pick up speed. Ten miles per hour, 15, 20, 25, 30, 35. When the train was only a few feet from me, I hit the deck, pancaking on the tracks below. I kept my eyes open. The sound was deafening. The tracks rattled, the crossties reverberated. It was the loudest noise I had ever felt. Forty-five tons of iron and steel passed over me. And I still had my nose. And toes.

The train had missed me by 6 inches and half a second. (That last sentence deserved an entire paragraph.)

I don't really know how this affected Tom Allison, but he did say, "You know, Shirk, I just had a feeling you were really going to do this. I kinda had that feeling from day one."

I think we both did.

The next morning I was more freaked out over this than any previous stunt. I couldn't even watch the video. Liz, who'd refused to stay for the live event, couldn't watch the tape, either. I didn't blame her.

There was little local coverage, again for fear others would try it. Interesting—if I had been killed, they'd have found a place on the front page. Trust me.

> When the train was only a few feet from me, I hit the deck, pancaking on the tracks below. I kept my eyes open. The sound was deafening. The tracks rattled, the crossties reverberated. It was the loudest noise I had ever felt. Forty-five tons of iron and steel passed over me. And I still had my nose. And toes.

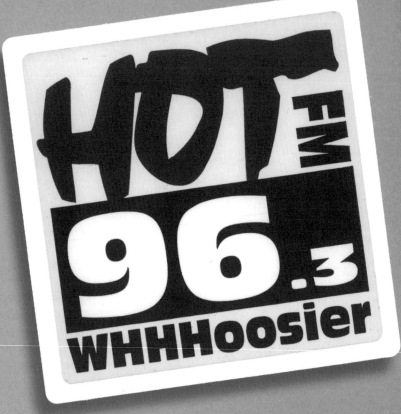

Climb to Success

IT WAS 1991. I had just orchestrated the purchase through the FCC of a license for a low-powered FM radio station, hocking half my life to do it. I was hoping to play rap and hip-hop music with a 3,000-watt signal. If people thought I was crazy before, you should have heard them now.

They told me I'd go broke. One radio analyst said: "Shirk will die promoting his new radio station." In one way, he was wrong. Which is why Dick Wolfsie and I are writing this book from my multimillion-dollar estate. In another way, he might have been correct, as you'll see.

One thing I did know. I needed to kick off my first morning on the air with a new escape or stunt that would create a little watercooler conversation and get some publicity in the media. I was pretty confident that my programming concept would work if people sampled the station's music.

A classic approach to promotion in radio is to tie your station frequency on the dial to some kind of giveaway or call-in. If you're 1070 on the AM dial, then, you might take the tenth and seventieth callers or give away $1,070 in a contest. Or $10.70, if you're really cheap, which Indianapolis station WIBC was at the time.

Taking this concept, which was probably invented by Marconi shortly after he created the radio itself, I decided I would climb the radio tower of my new station. It sat atop Indianapolis's then-highest structure, the Bank One Building. Because the number on the dial was 96.3, I planned to remain on top of the tower for nine hours, six minutes, and three seconds. I probably should have stayed on for ninety-six hours and three minutes, but if WIBC can give away $10.70, this was good enough for me.

I wasn't going to climb the whole building; I was Radio-Man, not Spider-Man. I planned to make my way to the top of the radio tower, some 250 feet above a hatch in the roof of the building. The tower had crossmembers, intended for people

> **I decided I would climb the radio tower of my new station. It sat atop Indianapolis's then-highest structure, the Bank One Building. Because the number on the dial was 96.3, I planned to remain on top of the tower for nine hours, six minutes, and three seconds.**

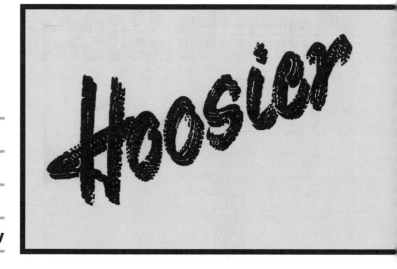

> I threw fashion to the wind and dressed in a ski outfit, mountain climbing boots, a wool hat, and a big old floppy black vinyl raincoat. This was probably the silliest I looked since I was sitting in a jockstrap in the Hamilton County Jail.

executing repairs. It wasn't executing I was afraid of. It was electrocuting.

When I awoke at 4:00 A.M. on Halloween—the morning of our sign-on—it was cold, damp, and dreary. Not a perfect day to climb or be seen climbing.

To make matters worse, ever since the White River swim several years earlier I had developed a dread of cold and wet weather. That 2-mile swim, you may recall, landed me in the hospital with pneumonia.

I threw fashion to the wind and dressed in a ski outfit, mountain climbing boots, a wool hat, and a big old floppy black vinyl raincoat. This was probably the silliest I looked since I was sitting in a jockstrap in the Hamilton County Jail. But I was a heck of a lot warmer. So far.

I reached the Bank One Building. I stepped out of the car and realized there was trouble. It was raining hard and the winds were whipping at 25 miles per hour, pretty gusty even for a gutsy guy like me. I knew that 1,000 feet up, this had *you're an idiot* written all over it.

I climbed the stairs to the roof of the building, where I met a couple of employees ready to assist me with the climb. Because I had no way to communicate with people below, we settled on a system of flags, yellow and red, to establish how things were proceeding. Yellow was essentially a green light (we couldn't find a green flag), but red meant "get your ass down here." I couldn't imagine a scenario where that would happen. Apparently I didn't have a very good imagination.

WHHH FM
INDY'S NEW
MUSIC MIX!
FM 96 DOT 3

I began climbing the
250-foot tower in a
driving rainstorm,
moving vertically
through the clouds.
The 25-mile-per-hour
wind swirled around
me, bending the
tower like a huge
pole-vaulting pole.

I began climbing the 250-foot tower in a driving rainstorm, moving vertically through the clouds. The 25-mile-per-hour wind swirled around me, bending the tower like a huge pole-vaulting pole. I had a vision of being catapulted into space and setting a new world record for first person to go into orbit without a rocket. Before that happened, however, I planted an American flag at the top of the tower.

One little secret. I did ultimately fasten myself with a safety line to the tower, but even so, the fear factor was intense. Much more so than with the helicopter, which had taken me 600 feet higher. Here, because the building provided perspective, there was a greater sense of height and more anxiety about falling.

As the tower continued to sway, I popped on my transistor radio to listen to my new station and get an update on how I was doing. They were on remote, covering the climb. The reception was perfect, by the way. Why not? I was 30 feet from the antenna.

My DJ was lamenting the fact that clouds had pretty much obscured the view. "WE KNOW HE'S UP THERE," he screamed. "BUT WHERE? WE CAN'T SEE HIM."

I wasn't happy about the lack of visibility, but I did think that the promotion would work. I fantasized thousands of people standing below, hoping to get a glimpse. If they got bored, maybe they'd go home and turn on their radio to 96.3. At the very least there would be reporters, TV cameras, the works.

Then the unthinkable. The weather started to clear. I

looked down and saw my colleagues waving the red flag. *"YOU'RE WAVING THE WRONG FLAG,"* I screamed. *"ARE YOU COLOR-BLIND, OR WHAT?"*

The red continued to wave, now more frantically. I could faintly hear them screaming. *"YA GOTTA COME DOWN. NOW. RIGHT NOW."*

Slowly and carefully I made my way down the tower, negotiating what had become a thin layer of ice on the cross-rails. The process was agonizingly slow because I had to continually reestablish the safety rope as I descended.

"What is going on?" I snapped when I got to the hatch.

"The Secret Service is in the building."

"You gotta be kidding. Why?"

I then found out what all the commotion was about. Vice President Dan Quayle had arrived in Indianapolis to give a speech. Where? In the same building I was dangling on top of. Lunatics on tops of buildings armed with pocket transistor radios were considered dangerous. I basically had been given two choices: Come down on my own slowly, or come down quickly with a bullet in my head. Okay, that's a bit of an exaggeration, but I still got the picture.

Waiting for me below was a United Press International reporter who thought the entire story was a stitch and wrote it up for the national press. Ironically, it was because of Quayle's visit that I got as much publicity as I did. The truth was that few people had come to the bank building, so the news story, which also appeared locally, gave me and the station a boost.

How big a boost? By the first rating book, 96.3, which we called Hoosier Hot 96, had cut into the ratings of both contemporary WZPL and urban WTLC, garnering a 5.1 share, the best first rating for any new Indiana radio station in thirty years. I felt like a kid again. But in one way, I felt like an old man. You see, I was wearing Depends, a precaution I took in case nature called while I was on the flag pole. Which it did.

What was next? I was going from 1,000 feet up to 6 feet below. Little did I know what was in store for me.

On December 9, 1991, at the age of forty-six, when some of my buddies were becoming grandparents, I found myself in the delivery room watching the birth of my daughter, Maxine. Becoming a father for the first time is almost as scary as putting your head in a bag with a rattlesnake. And I even kept my eyes open.

By the first rating book, 96.3, which we called Hoosier Hot 96, had cut into the ratings of both contemporary WZPL and urban WTLC, garnering a 5.1 share, the best first rating for any new Indiana radio station in thirty years.

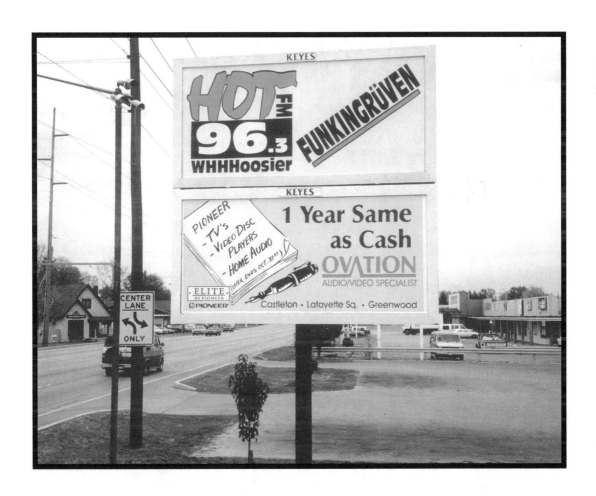

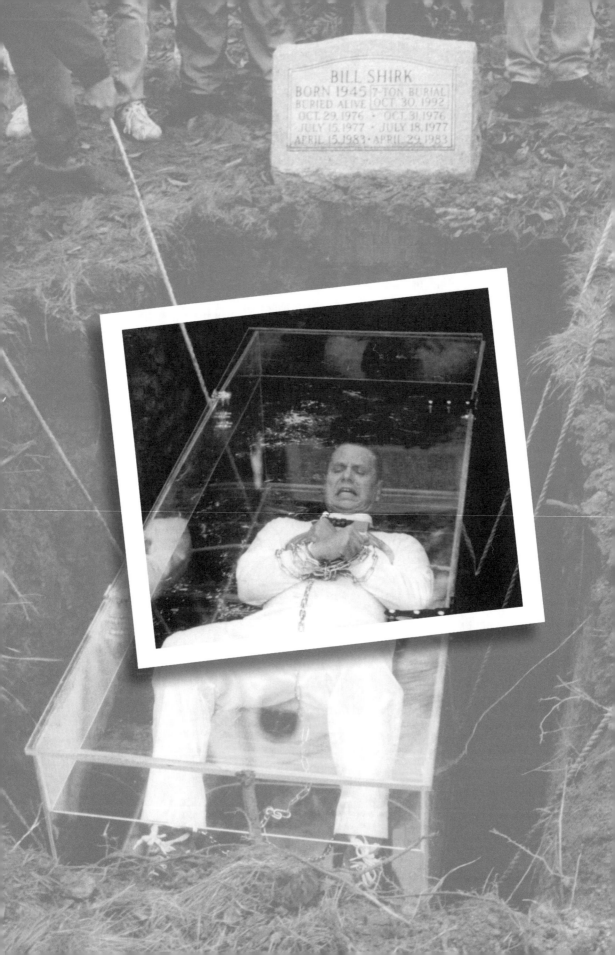

Grave Consequences

ON HALLOWEEN 1990 IN CALIFORNIA, an escape artist named Joe Burris was buried in a Plexiglas coffin under tons of dirt and cement while chained and handcuffed. After he was completely dug up, he was completely dead.

I had been doing escapes for more than fifteen years and I knew this was a pretty good indication that something had gone wrong. But I liked the idea of the escape and decided to call the popular TV show *A Current Affair* to suggest to them that I could do a similar escape with a better result.

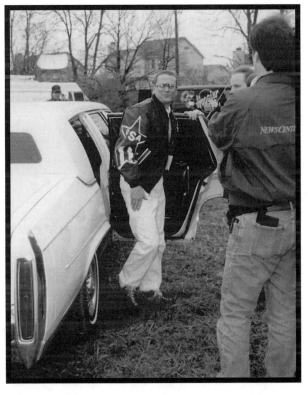

I promised them I wouldn't die and they promised me $5,000. At the time it seemed like a pretty good deal (as long as we both kept our word), though the truth was that I was not, at that point, quite sure how Burris did it. Or more precisely, how he didn't do it.

I was about to learn. The hard way. The way I learned almost everything.

I had made to order several Plexiglas coffins, not a stocked item at most mortuaries, and experimented with the amount of weight each coffin could sustain. Using a backhoe to incrementally add dirt and a truck to add the cement pretty much convinced me that doing this escape as Burris had done it was truly suicide. Every time the coffin collapsed, I nearly felt my chest collapse with it. It was almost humbling.

Joe's mistake was not realizing that digging your way out of that much dead weight was impossible. He lacked a method to bypass some of the dirt and cement and still get to the top. He hadn't given the escape very much thought. Been there, done that. Sound familiar?

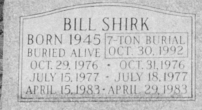

BILL SHIRK
BORN 1945
BURIED ALIVE
OCT. 29, 1976 · OCT. 31, 1976
JULY 15, 1977 · JULY 18, 1977
APRIL 15, 1983 · APRIL 29, 1983
7-TON BURIAL
OCT. 30, 1992

My major goal was to survive the stunt (I didn't care so much how I got out), but I did not want it to be a trick.

My major goal was to survive the stunt (I didn't care so much how I got out), but I did not want it to be a trick. The public needed to know that I was, indeed, underground and that seven tons of dirt and cement had been poured on top of me.

I needed a technique to survive the ordeal, not an illusion to persuade people I was in the coffin when I wasn't. That's an important distinction. It's why both Joe and I used the Plexiglas coffin and not a wooden one. That way, the audience could see that I was really in the coffin.

I realized that I would need help getting out. This would not detract from what I saw as the most dramatic and important part of the escape: my survival.

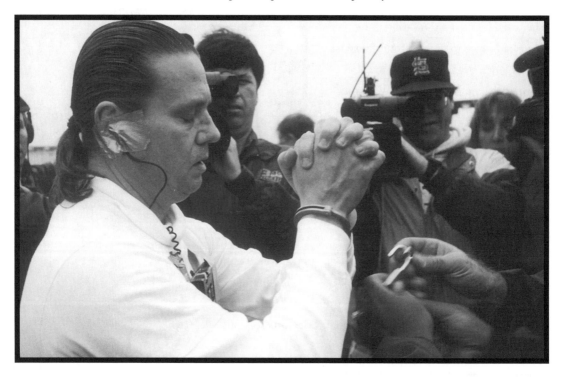

The answer was a good backhoe operator, one who recognized the importance of digging carefully and not dislodging my head. I found a guy who had made quite a name for himself in town by doing a TV commercial in which he'd attached a wooden match to the backhoe and then effortlessly rubbed it across a slab of concrete to strike it and light it.

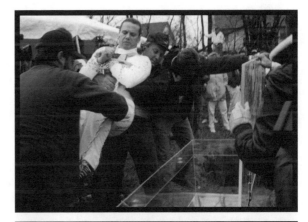

He was perfect.

Now I needed a plan of escape from the coffin. While it was true that the backhoe would be digging me out, I also needed to dig up. And you can't dig up when you are buried in dirt and cement. I needed a method to avoid being crushed and a way to sustain normal breathing during the escape period.

On Halloween, the day of the escape, every local TV station was there as well as media from around the country and even some from Europe. Everything was going according to plan.

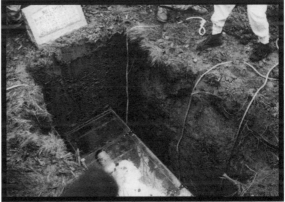

Almost everything.

When I examined the hole in the ground that we had dug the night before, something troubled me. The hole had not been excavated to my specifications—specifications that took into account how much dirt you could put back in the hole and how much pressure that would exert on the sides and top of the coffin. This hole was too big. That would throw off my calculated predictions of when the glass case would crack and cave in. I knew that it would, I just wanted an idea when. That would help me plan my escape before being crushed to death.

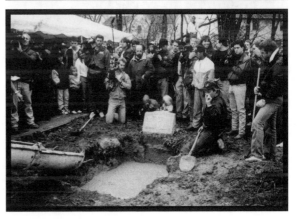

That wasn't all. It had rained the night before. The hole was filled with water, and the dirt to cover the coffin was now mud. Mud weighs more than dirt. Much, much more. I had

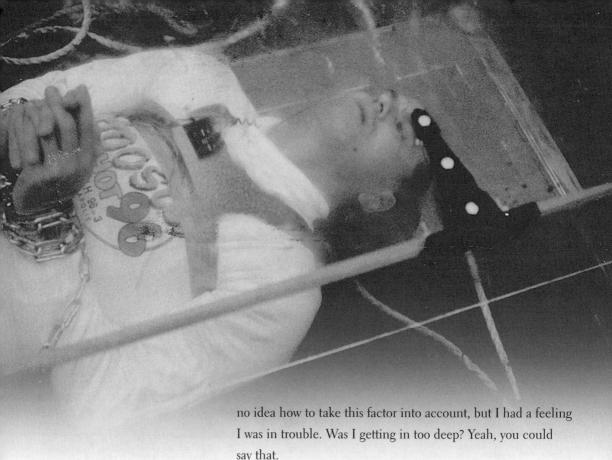

no idea how to take this factor into account, but I had a feeling I was in trouble. Was I getting in too deep? Yeah, you could say that.

The phrase *chicken out* was not in my vocabulary. *Stretch it out* was in my vocabulary, but not *chicken out*. I didn't mind building suspense, but I wasn't going to back out.

As you'll see, however, backing out is exactly how I did it.

I arrived in a limo, dressed in traditional red, white, and blue garb. Along with the media, I had an ambulance and two paramedics standing by. I wasn't taking any chances. (Oh, the hell I wasn't.)

The escape began. A police officer, Ricky Clark, put me in two sets of handcuffs, a pair of leg cuffs, and several feet of chain, just as in the jailbreak. I had forgotten to mention that little detail, hadn't I? Hey, I'm a modest guy.

I was placed in the coffin and the box padlocked. As the box was lowered into the ground, my assistants carefully packed the dirt around it—important because the dirt supported the sides of the coffin and sealed the air inside.

I saw the shovels of dirt beginning to cover the coffin. Suddenly everything went black. Total darkness. The good news was that I could begin extricating myself from the

I saw the shovels of dirt beginning to cover the coffin. Suddenly everything went black. Total darkness.

restraints, a task easily accomplished by removing a "key" that I had hidden in my shoes. I had actually been searched by police for any concealed tools, but they'd never looked in my shoes. Nowadays they even look in your shoes at the airport.

I was out of all the restraints in minutes. But that was never my concern.

I heard creaking. Creaking was a bad thing to hear. It meant something was about to break apart. I expected that. I also expected that the dirt now being layered on top of the coffin would tend to gravitate toward my feet when the coffin broke. Same for the cement that would follow. I knew this from previous experience, and so had instructed my assistants on how to properly disperse the weight to ensure this result.

The coffin was still creaking. One creak was near my head, and I knew that if the coffin split there I was in danger of the shards cutting my throat or decapitating me. That's what happened to Joe Burris.

And now you will learn the real secret of my escape, never told before. The bottom of the Plexiglas coffin was sectioned. I was able to remove about a third of the flooring and use that

> **The coffin was still creaking. One creak was near my head, and I knew that if the coffin split there I was in danger of the shards cutting my throat or decapitating me. That's what happened to Joe Burris.**

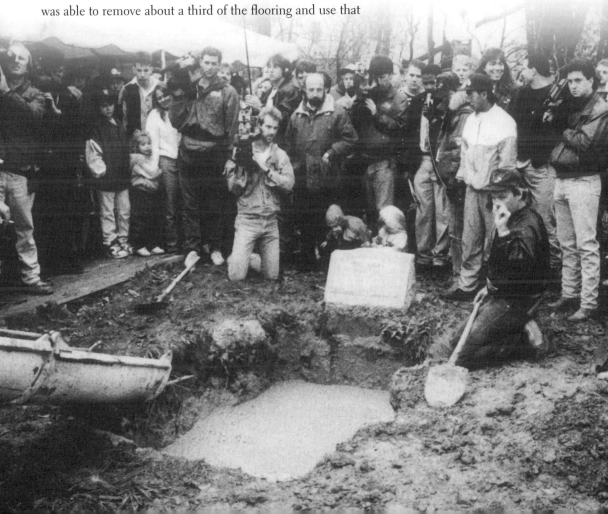

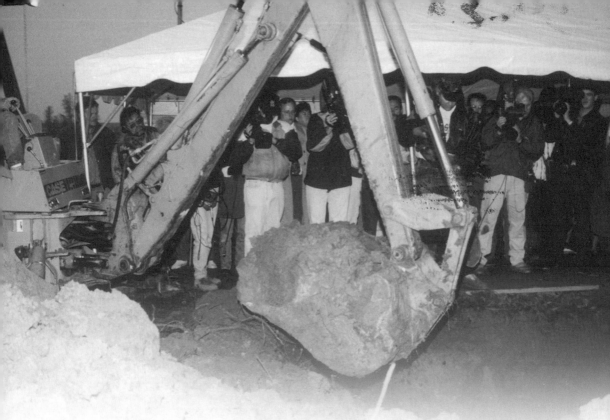

At five-forty the cement was layered in, and within a few minutes the coffin collapsed.

slab as a barrier—a barrier that, when wedged into the floor at a forty-five-degree angle, would protect me from all the wet dirt and cement that could potentially crush or smother me. Essentially, I was hiding behind it, like a knight's shield.

While making this adjustment in the coffin, I added a bit of suspense to the proceedings by feigning second thoughts and a feeling of dread. At five-fifteen I asked that they postpone the cement for a few minutes until I gathered my wits.

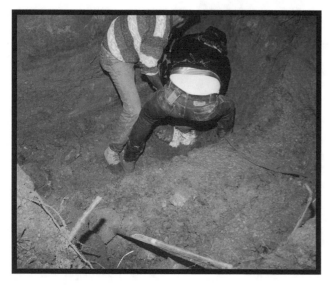

Of course, my real motive in stalling was to secure the barricade and make sure that the local news would be at its peak hour during the collapse of the coffin.

At five-forty the cement was layered in, and within a few minutes the coffin collapsed. Everyone thought I was dead. My escape technique worked like a charm, but by the time the backhoe had reached me and the media saw my hand reach through the dirt, it was almost twenty-two minutes.

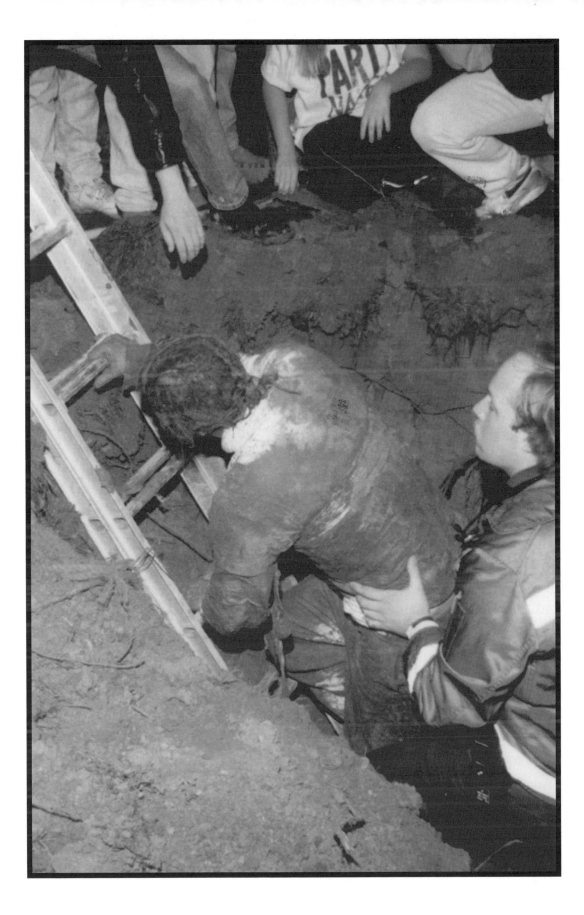

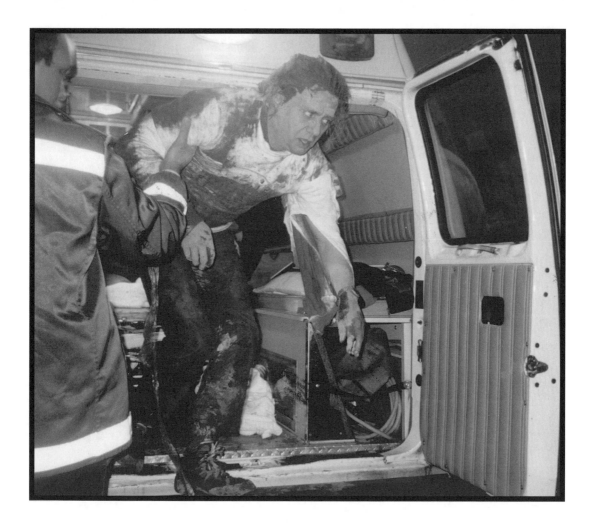

I was pulled from the grave covered with mud and cement. I had been breathing my own carbon dioxide for the last several minutes and was delirious. They placed an oxygen mask on me and I recuperated for quite a while in the ambulance.

The local TV stations had thought I was dead. They had actually broken into the national news with updates. *A Current Affair* aired the spectacle a week later.

I had done what I had proposed. How I did it was not really the issue. I had a very ingenious technique. It wasn't a trick. I was really underground, buried under seven tons of dirt and cement.

In some ways, this was the perfect escape. Why? Because everyone thought I was dead.

But I was alive to talk about it.

They placed an oxygen mask on me and I recuperated for quite a while in the ambulance.

My Husband, the Escape Artist

By Liz Poorman

I was twenty-four years old and a waitress in a local discotheque. It wasn't unusual for guys to try to pick me up. But it was unusual for a guy to wrap a $20 bill around his business card and give it to me.

And this was not just any business card; it was a mini résumé, listing all Bill's accomplishments beginning with schoolteacher and including DJ, escape artist, and racecar driver. Quite frankly, the list did intrigue me, except the part about being a notary public. I guess Bill was covering all his bases. There might have been a woman somewhere who was into stuff like that.

I think most women would have been turned off by such an approach, but my dad, whom I loved very much, was a kind of daredevil and also sought the limelight. He was no escape artist, but he was an adventurer and loved living on the edge. I think I needed something like that in my life. I wasn't the kind of girl to marry a dentist.

Although Bill and I dated for many years before getting married, marriage was not among his many escapes. During our entire relationship, I have never once asked Bill not to go through with an escape.

There were stunts that troubled me (like the shark tank); one or two I chose not to see in person (like the cement burial); but never, ever did I ask Bill not to go through with one. That's who Bill is and I've trusted him. Despite what people have said, Bill does not have a death wish. He has had too much to live for. Like me.

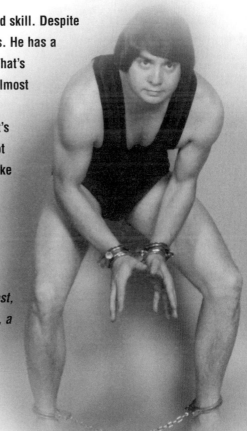

Bill Shirk's life has been a great combination of luck and skill. Despite a few lean years, I knew he would be successful in business. He has a great radio mind, but he doesn't focus well on everything. That's where I come in. I'm his personal assistant. I take care of almost everything else in our lives.

In many ways Bill and I are exact opposites. I think that's why the marriage works. If we were the same—well, I'm not sure a marriage like that could last very long. Two people like Bill Shirk could not live in the same house.

If I walked into a bar and someone asked what my husband, Bill Shirk, did for a living, here's what I'd say:

After one martini: *Oh, my husband is in radio.*

After two martinis: *My husband is an escape artist.*

After three martinis: *My husband is the kindest, sweetest, most generous person in the world. He's a wonderful father, a loyal husband, and a kind and generous employer.*

After four martinis: *Bill who?*

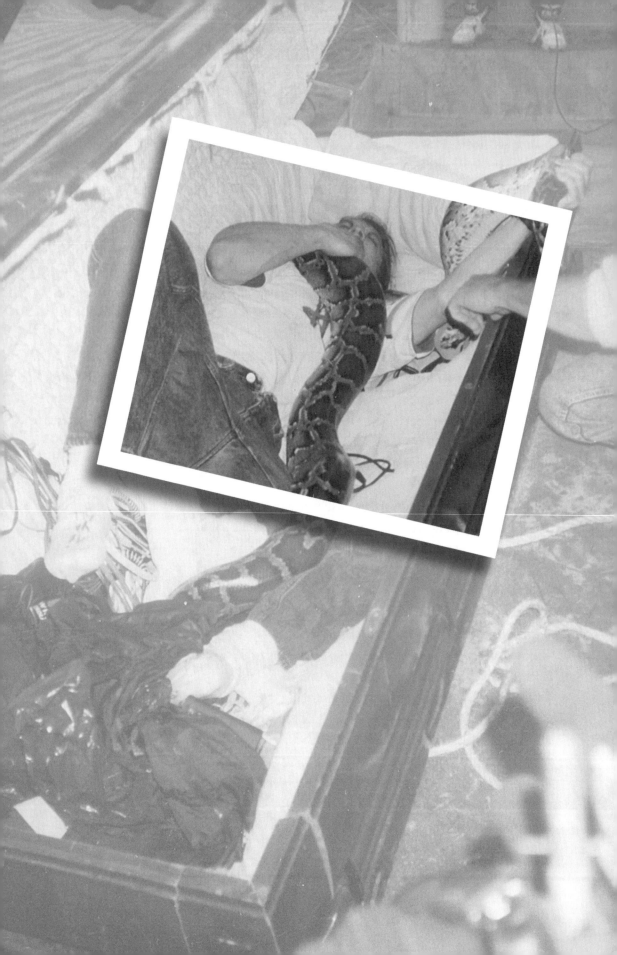

Spider Man

I WAS SLOWLY COMING TO A RATHER UNSETTLING
conclusion: I was a bigger hit when I screwed up than when I
was successful. When the rope suspending me over Orca didn't
burn in two, I got on national TV to redo the stunt—this time
over hungry sharks. Then the seven-ton burial, which did not
live up to any of my expectations, garnered international
publicity and culminated in an appearance on a slew of network
shows, the Disney Channel, and the Discovery Channel. Even
Montel Williams invited me to be on his talk show.

Williams never even
mentioned that I had failed
to climb out of the coffin
successfully. He didn't care.
No one cared. I had escaped
death. That's what this was
all about. If I did something
crazy and survived, that's
what counted. Okay, fine.

About this time my
business ventures took on a
new complexity. New FCC
rules allowed me to
purchase additional radio

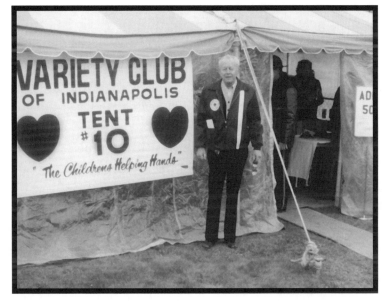

stations in the Indianapolis market, as well as a low-powered
TV station. Convinced that I needed to expand, I pursued this
idea, but my initial investors were not happy with this decision.
They wanted my undivided attention on our current properties
and were so put off by my ambition that they threatened a
lawsuit to prevent me from expanding.

I approached Bill Mays, a local businessman and
entrepreneur, who agreed to buy out my investors for $3.4
million. They had nothing to complain about. They made out
like bandits, netting more than three million bucks in less than
three years. After the buyout Mays and I purchased two
additional FM stations and a TV station. What was I doing? I

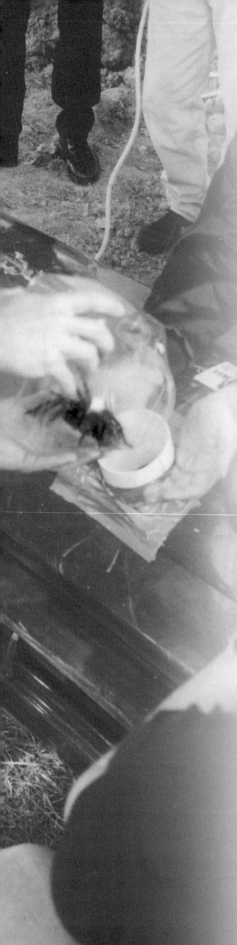

now owed millions. The entire situation would become a programming and coordination nightmare, but my old instinct told me that to kick off my new stations I needed another escape with a unique twist to get me some media attention.

About this time an inner-city Scout leader asked me to assist the Scouts in obtaining camping equipment. How could we raise $5,000 for the Scouts and promote my new properties at the same time? I could bury myself one more time. How about for ninety-six hours? Sure, why not? And I'd be dug up Halloween on the sixty-eighth anniversary of Houdini's death.

I had no intention of being down there all alone. Of course, no sane human being wanted to accompany me, so I opted for a couple of my nephew's pets: a 15-foot Burmese python and a Venezuelan Goliath bird-eating spider—not only poisonous, but, like a rottweiler, a creature with a less-than-stellar record for congeniality. The spider was also somewhat like a miniature poodle. Because that's how big it was. Almost.

The morning of the burial, I felt pretty good. I was using my old coffin—the one I'd previously been buried in for two weeks with a slew of rats—which, ironically, offered some comfort. A long pipe was inserted in the coffin lid so that the necessary electrical wires could be strung into the coffin. I would also be getting air and water through the pipe, which extended from the surface to the inside of the box through the lid. The inside of the coffin had lighting, a TV camera, and a phone system. Needless to say, I was not looking forward to this, but I was ready.

The drama began way before I was lowered into the coffin. The coffin had not only a lid, but also a kind of hinged door on the side that could be opened like the flap of a breadbox, but from the bottom. As a result, the media could see and record exactly what was happening. Once I was on my back, the python was inserted in the tube, and it slithered into the coffin and wrapped itself around me. Then came the itsy, bitsy spider down the water spout. (This spider was certainly not related to the one from that cute little song. That spider didn't eat birds.)

By the way, I did *not* have a particular dread of spiders, but there is something almost instinctive in humans that finds

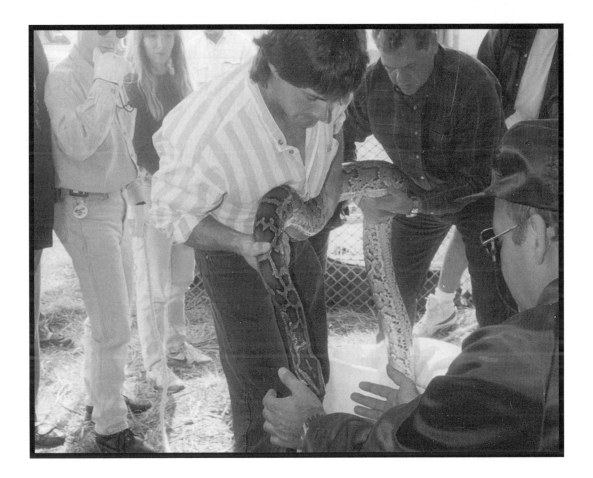

them repulsive. I was beginning to understand this. The spider plopped right on my face and just sat there. On top of my right eye. The coffin lid was closed. The flap shut and the box was lowered into the earth.

A minute later my brain was throbbing. It was pure agony. The spider's legs had tiny quills and they had become embedded in my face, leaving behind spinelike slivers. I thought my head would explode.

The coffin hit bottom, and I heard the crew beginning to cover the wooden box with dirt. I quickly unraveled the python from my chest and safely sealed him in my discarded pants as I had done in previous burials.

Meanwhile, the bird-eating spider had perched himself on one of the walls of the coffin. He was just sitting there, like a damn clock on the wall. What was he doing? Was he thinking about getting vicious? I was a sitting duck. A duck is a bird, isn't it? I had no idea what to expect.

Once I was on my back, the python was inserted in the tube, and it slithered into the coffin and wrapped itself around me.

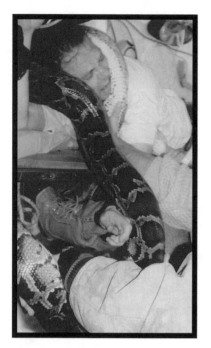

A large crowd would gather above. Bystanders could talk to me on the phone or watch me on the TV monitor a direct feed from the TV camera in the coffin. In some cases skeptics would question if I was really down there, at which time I would request through the speaker system that they lower some water to me so that I could get a drink. Minutes later I requested that the skeptic pull the rope up to retrieve the empty bottle.

But I didn't send the bottle back empty. I used the bottle to piss in. Dick Wolfsie and I have tried to find a nice way to say this, and that's the best we could come up with. Yeah, I relieved myself in the bottle. (Yes, that's better.) And the crowd loved it. Every time that bottle reached ground level, I could hear the laughter. I'd have done it more often, but I was in a coffin, not a saloon.

I had been underground close to sixty-nine hours when I awoke from a brief nap. I found myself covered in sweat. My chest felt tight. I was having difficulty breathing. And I was in total darkness. What was happening? I fumbled for the flashlight, but couldn't find it. Then the old standby. I reached into my sock and pulled out a book of matches. I tried to light the first one. Nothing. Maybe it was damp. The second. Still nothing. Three, four, and five. Zilch. The answer was painfully obvious: There was no oxygen in the coffin. I was slowly suffocating.

I panicked. You haven't heard me use that word before in this book. It was the middle of the night. There was no one above. No one to help me. Everyone had gone home. Even if there were folks up there, it would take forty-five minutes to dig me out. How much air did I have left? I didn't have a clue.

I fumbled around in the dark, grabbing for the sides of the box. Suddenly I felt a sweatshirt in my hand—a sweatshirt that I'd inadvertently shoved into the opening of the pipe that connected to the surface. The sweatshirt had stopped the flow of air. I was breathing my own carbon dioxide. I had apparently disconnected the electric plug as well, probably kicking it in my sleep.

Annoyed at my own stupidity, but pleased that I had solved the problem, I patiently maintained as much calm as I

Then the old standby. I reached into my sock and pulled out a book of matches. I tried to light the first one. Nothing. Maybe it was damp. The second. Still nothing. Three, four, and five. Zilch. The answer was painfully obvious: There was no oxygen in the coffin. I was slowly suffocating.

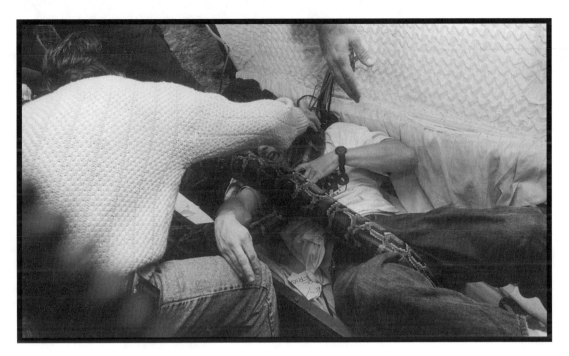

could, breathing methodically and sucking the air from the
pipe. I slowly began to feel better.

I had kept up pretty good communication with the outside
world, chatting with radio hosts from across the country. Pretty
standard stuff with the predictable questions: How are you? Are
you sleeping? What are you eating? Are you bored? Do you
want to get out? How do you go to the bathroom? Are you
scared? What's that snake doing? How's the spider?

Then a fascinating call. A talk-show host from WJR in
Detroit told me that a professor—and an expert in
spiders—at the University of Detroit had been
following the story and was aghast. Apparently, this
guy had a few of these bird-eating spiders himself
and was just astounded that I had locked myself in
a coffin with one. "These are vicious," he told the
DJ. "This Shirk guy better watch out."

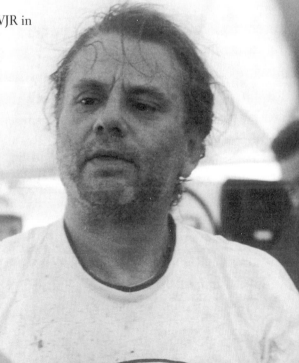

The DJ and I arranged for an interview with
the professor, whose concern would lend some
credibility to my stunt, I thought, or at the
very least make it sound creepier. I was
looking forward to the interview, but I
wasn't sure I could give the professor much
insight into the spider's behavior. That sucker

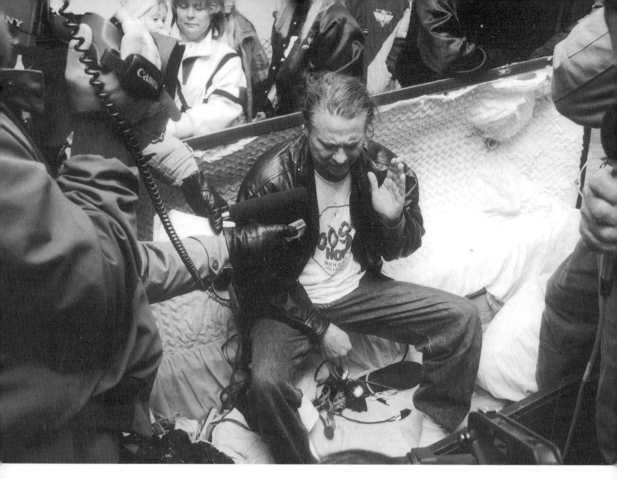

It was Halloween, ninety-six hours after the burial. Time to be exhumed. The wooden platform we had placed above the coffin had become wedged in the rough box in which the coffin sat. They couldn't open the lid.

was still just flat against the wall. Hadn't moved in seventy-two hours. I reached up and gently nudged him, half afraid he'd jump and sink his little quills into my face again.

I touched him again. I gently prodded him. I even screamed at him. Nothing. Why? Because he was dead, that's why. And why was he dead? He must have died when the oxygen level had dropped in the coffin. The spider was a big wimp. Hey, I was still alive and I needed a lot more oxygen than he did. A couple of hours later, I spoke with the professor. I never told him the spider was dead. I just said we hadn't paid much attention to one another. "He kinda keeps to himself," I noted. And that was true.

It was Halloween, ninety-six hours after the burial. Time to be exhumed. The wooden platform we had placed above the coffin had become wedged in the rough box in which the coffin sat. They couldn't open the lid. Extricating me required the use of a circular saw. Sawdust flew and the sound of the blades punctuated the air. It was just the touch of drama I needed. I wished I had thought of it on my own. (Actually, I did. That was the plan from the beginning.)

At my request, the coffin was lifted and placed in the middle of the waiting crowd. I jumped out of the box, the snake draped around my neck and shoulders, and began dancing and whooping it up. I was on an adrenaline high. The crowd responded in kind. It was like a big fraternity party. Everyone seemed to be having fun. Except the spider.

Two cheeseburgers and a milk shake later, I tried to assess just how successful the escape had been. It went off exactly as planned and we had raised the necessary $5,000 for the Scouts, but some of the media had boycotted me, claiming they would not assist me in promoting my huge ego.

If I had suffocated and died, they'd have covered the story. Success was killing me.

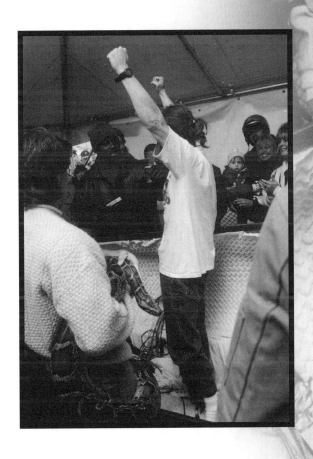

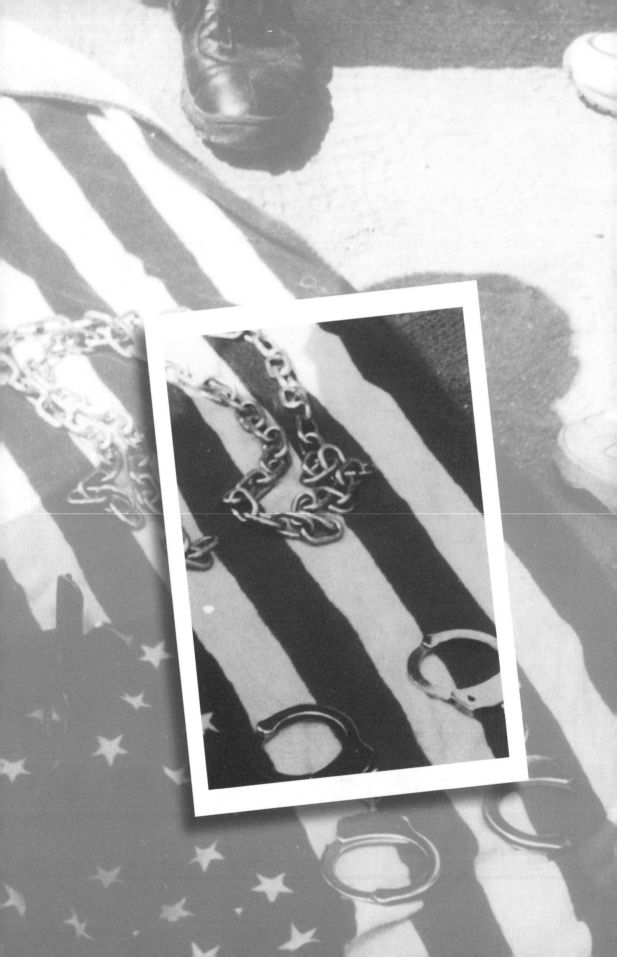

The Heart of an Escapologist

EVER SINCE I WAS TWELVE YEARS OLD, I have known I was a walking time bomb. In 1957 a doctor told my parents I had a heart murmur, the result of a faulty aortic valve. Since there was little they could do in those days, the doctor restricted most of my athletic activity, including bike riding. For a hyper kid who loved doing what every kid loves, this was devastating.

Later, in high school, I pretty much said the heck with it, and my parents even allowed me to compete in athletic activities. I lettered in several sports, but I always knew it was just a matter of time. Maybe this is when I first took a different view of my own mortality. I think it made me stronger. And less afraid of death in the context of performing a daredevil stunt.

Over the years I did not obsess over this, but I did go for regular checkups to be sure there was no change. I always knew that someday, something would have to be done.

It was now 1997. I didn't need bacon, sweet rolls, and pizza to aggravate my heart condition. I had three FM radio stations and a TV station. I also owed $4 million. And I wasn't feeling well. In fact, I hadn't felt very good since the seven-ton burial years earlier. I was easily fatigued. Something wasn't right.

The doctor confirmed my worst fear: It was time to replace the aortic valve that had served me pretty well for fifty-two years, the very age at which Houdini died. The valve had calcified, reducing the size of the opening, and was pumping

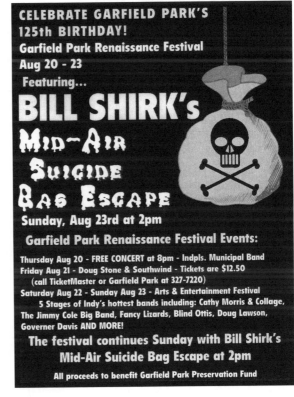

CELEBRATE GARFIELD PARK'S 125th BIRTHDAY!
Garfield Park Renaissance Festival
Aug 20 - 23
Featuring...
BILL SHIRK's
MID-AIR SUICIDE BAG ESCAPE
Sunday, Aug 23rd at 2pm
Garfield Park Renaissance Festival Events:
Thursday Aug 20 - FREE CONCERT at 8pm - Indpls. Municipal Band
Friday Aug 21 - Doug Stone & Southwind - Tickets are $12.50
(call TicketMaster or Garfield Park at 327-7220)
Saturday Aug 22 - Sunday Aug 23 - Arts & Entertainment Festival
5 Stages of Indy's hottest bands including: Cathy Morris & Collage,
The Jimmy Cole Big Band, Fancy Lizards, Blind Ottis, Doug Lawson,
Governer Davis AND MORE!
The festival continues Sunday with Bill Shirk's
Mid-Air Suicide Bag Escape at 2pm
All proceeds to benefit Garfield Park Preservation Fund

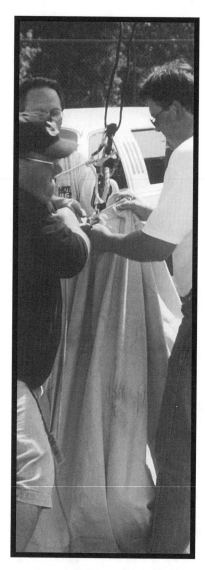

only 35 percent of the oxygenated blood back into my system. I needed open-heart surgery. That in itself was a bit scary, but not as troubling as what they planned to do: The doctors wanted to replace my aortic valve with either a pig valve or a plastic one.

Both procedures had a pretty good track record, but the implications for me were troubling. Postoperative, patients of this technique were required to take for the rest of their lives a blood-thinning drug called Coumadin. This would have meant the end of my escape career. Any cut, scrape, or wound could have a catastrophic effect on me.

"You must find another way," I told the doctor. "There must be an alternative."

Apparently, there was. The Ross method used a person's own pulmonary valve to replace the aorta. The pulmonary valve, which is not utilized as much as the aorta, is replaced by a cadaver's valve.

The technique was not foolproof (that phrase keeps coming up with me, doesn't it?). Arnold Schwarzenegger had undergone a similar procedure and had experienced serious complications, requiring a second operation with a more traditional approach. In addition, I was informed that this particular method was really intended for younger people because when successful, the valve could last for seventy-five years, which was kind of a waste on a guy of fifty-plus. They didn't say it quite like that, but I got the picture.

The operation was scheduled for Halloween. As you know from reading this book so far, I love to do life-threatening things on Halloween. Would I once again escape death? Houdini hadn't. He died at 52.

I asked the doctor if we could videotape the surgery and if I could have a snake around my neck. For a brief moment, he thought I was serious. What about you?

The surgery was ill-timed in many ways. Things were abuzz back at the radio and TV stations, and I had multiple duties as owner, programmer, and air personality for four different properties. Thank God for virtual radio, which allowed me to preproduce dozens of shows to air while I was under the knife and recuperating.

I asked the doctor if we could videotape the surgery and if I could have a snake around my neck. For a brief moment, he thought I was serious.

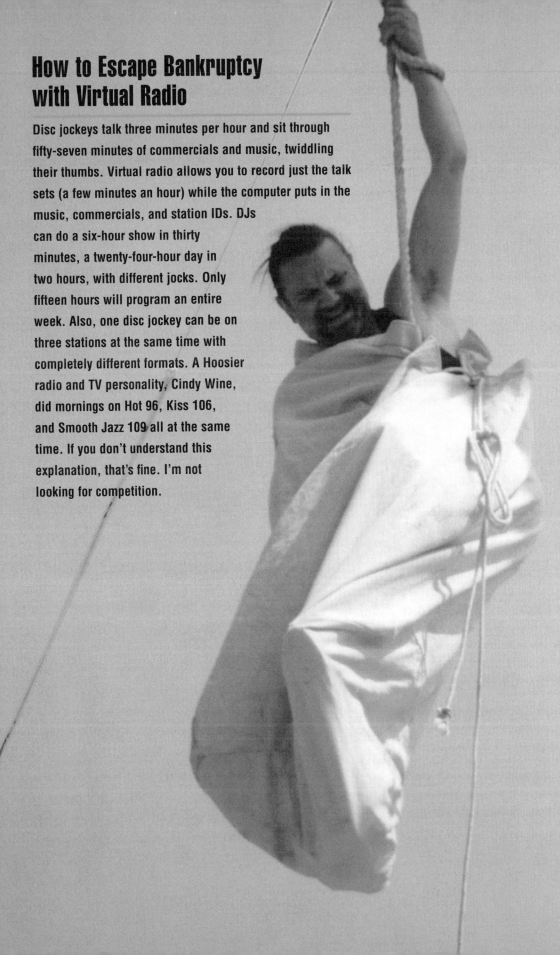

How to Escape Bankruptcy with Virtual Radio

Disc jockeys talk three minutes per hour and sit through fifty-seven minutes of commercials and music, twiddling their thumbs. Virtual radio allows you to record just the talk sets (a few minutes an hour) while the computer puts in the music, commercials, and station IDs. DJs can do a six-hour show in thirty minutes, a twenty-four-hour day in two hours, with different jocks. Only fifteen hours will program an entire week. Also, one disc jockey can be on three stations at the same time with completely different formats. A Hoosier radio and TV personality, Cindy Wine, did mornings on Hot 96, Kiss 106, and Smooth Jazz 109 all at the same time. If you don't understand this explanation, that's fine. I'm not looking for competition.

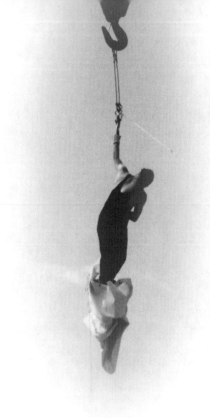

When I awoke from surgery, I experienced pure panic. A tube was down my throat, and my hands were tied so that I could not rip out the device. For a guy who made a career out of being tied up and chained, this reaction may seem a little out of character. Nevertheless, I was almost out of control until Liz came into the room, had the tube removed, and calmed me down.

I was back at work in three weeks, far from the original prognosis of several months.

I was feeling pretty good, but I needed to convince myself and others that this was not Bill Shirk's last hurrah. I needed a new stunt. Something different. Something I could not have physically managed before the surgery. Something I could put my new heart into.

I remembered a stunt that was suggested to me by a clown. Many clowns have suggested stunts to me, but this was a real clown, like in a circus. He had followed my career and suggested that I be handcuffed and chained inside a bag. The top of the bag would be tied, then a block and tackle attached to it. The bag would be hoisted upside down, 40 feet into the air. Then the bag would fall to the ground. People would think I was dead in the bag, but then I'd reveal myself from the top of the arena. Basically, the trick was not unlike the original train illusion. To the audience it would appear as though I was getting in the bag, but I would actually duck behind it and go down the stairs.

"Hey, that's a magic act," I told him, "I'm an escape artist"—which is a distinction too subtle for your average clown. I told him that I thought I could escape from the bag and have the bag quickly fall while I hung on to the supporting rope. The clown just smiled at me. Since the smile was painted on his face, I'm not sure what he was really thinking.

For years I thought about this stunt, convinced there was a way to do it. I figured that once I freed myself from the handcuffs and chains, I could wriggle my hand through the hole in the bag and grab the supporting cable. I would untie the bag where it was connected to the rope and kick the bag off. The bag would fall, and I would be suspended in air,

I was feeling pretty good, but I needed to convince myself and others that this was not Bill Shirk's last hurrah. I needed a new stunt. Something different. Something I could not have physically managed before the surgery. Something I could put my new heart into.

hanging on for dear life. The stunt takes incredible strength because you have to manipulate your weight and the bag against gravity while holding on with one hand. It was a true circus act. I knew I could do it.

And I did in 1998. On Halloween, of course, at Garfield Park in Indianapolis. I proved to the world and myself that a little open-heart surgery would not deter me from remaining active and keeping my legend alive. Once again, the local media shunned me, but more than 1,000 people saw the stunt. Actually many more saw or heard it. I had my three radio stations and TV station cover it.

I was back in the game.

I proved to the world and myself that a little open-heart surgery would not deter me from remaining active and keeping my legend alive.

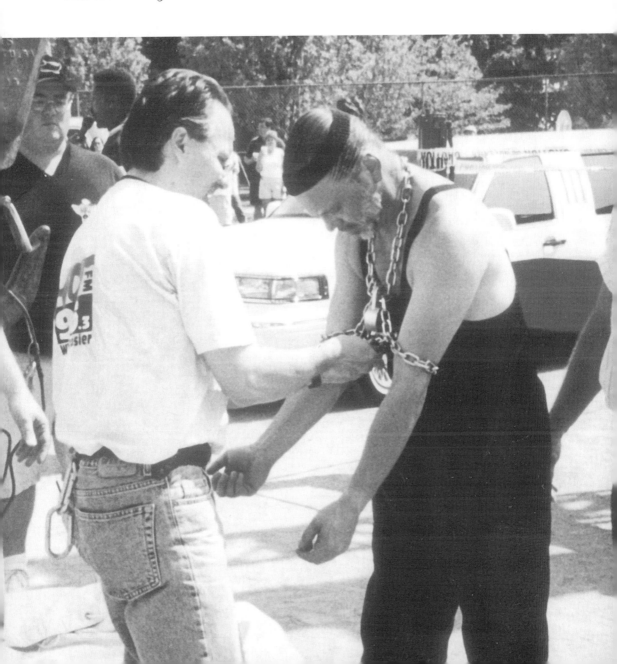

FOR IMMEDIATE RELEASE - August, 2000

To Be Broadcast 8:05pm(Eastern) Aug. 30 on TBS

Ripley's Believe It or Not!

FEATURING

BILL SHIRK - "The World's Greatest Escape Artist"

Hanging 60 feet upside down by his ankles, bound by 3 regulation police straitjackets, and a 15 foot, 150 pound Albino Burmese Python wrapped around his neck and body...

BILL SHIRK

...General Manager of Radio One, Indianapolis (WHHH-FM, WBKS-FM, WYJZ-FM & WAV TV-53) will perform this escape on the World-Wide Television show "Ripley's Believe It Or Not" on TBS.

This program is scheduled to be broadcast at 8:05pm(Eastern) Wednesday, August 30, 2000.

Bill Shirk has held 8 Guinness World Records.
His list of accomplishments include:

- Fastest Straitjacket Escape (4.52 sec.)
- Live burials with 14ft pythons, rats, spiders & rattlesnakes
- World Record Helicopter Escape (1610ft)
- The Great Train Escape
- Aquatic Death Trap (13 piranha)
- World Record Jailbreak

- Acapulco Cliff Jumps
- 7-Ton Dirt-Cement Burial
- Orca the Killer Whale Escape
- Locked in a Crystal Casket (13 scorpions)
- World Record Upsidedown Straitjacket Escape (7.2 sec.)

And the list goes on...

Bill Shirk is available for telephone interviews. Contact him at Hoosier Radio & TV (317) 293-9600

Believe It or Not

I WAS STILL ON A HIGH from the mid-air suicide bag escape, convinced that my strength was returning and that, even at fifty-plus, I still had more than a few escapes left in me.

I had become a workaholic with three radio stations and a TV station, and I was finally worth more money than I owed. My ship had not come in, but it was steaming toward the harbor. It was only a matter of time.

Then a call from *Ripley's Believe It or Not*, the TV show on TBS. I had always been wary of ties with them. In order to maintain my professional status, I needed to avoid the obvious stigma of being a freak or carnie—a label that pretty much went with the stories that the Ripley's folks did on TV and in their books.

But ironically my boyhood had been rich with circus and carnival experiences. My own dad, being in charge of the Delaware County Fair, had booked many acts that were clearly in the sideshow category. In addition, Houdini himself paid his dues doing the carnie circuit, attracting crowds and building a reputation that lead ultimately to financial success.

Not unlike what I did with ABC Sports, I gave the Ripley's people a list of three daredevil ideas and let them choose. Here were the choices. Read carefully, for the menu has changed:

1. Be locked in a crystal casket with thirteen poisonous scorpions while wearing two straitjackets. And escape.
2. Be tied in 25 feet of rope while hanging upside down with my head in a bag with a rattlesnake. And escape.
3. Be placed in three straitjackets with a 15-foot, 150-pound, albino Burmese python around my neck and body, hoisted into the air by my feet from a crane. And escape.

I wasn't thrilled about number one and I was kinda praying they wouldn't pick number two. The rattlesnake we had used in the circus escape had died and apparently Battson was now fresh out of sweethearts, so I wasn't sure what snake we would use.

> I had become a workaholic with three radio stations and a TV station, and I was finally worth more money than I owed. My ship had not come in, but it was steaming toward the harbor. It was only a matter of time.

The Ripley's people picked number three, though, which was a bit of a relief, except for one small problem. Actually, a long problem—15 feet long. How do you get a snake to Hollywood, California? The law was pretty clear: *You can't . . .* unless you have a special permit, which required red tape longer than the snake. Finally we arranged to ship him via U.S. air cargo. All this is a ticklish procedure because we were dealing with an expensive reptile prone to pneumonia if not kept warm. Battson told me that if the snake died, he'd be crushed. Of course, if the snake lived, I'd be crushed.

Battson told me that if the snake died, he'd be crushed. Of course, if the snake lived, I'd be crushed.

I guess I could have found a snake in California. There were plenty of them. I know, I tried to sell my film there.

The snake arrived ahead of us in California, but the Ripley's people apparently did not want to have any contact with my reptilian friend. Instead of meeting us at the airport, they simply left us a van so we could drive ourselves to the hotel.

It was a gorgeous hotel, and the room had a bathtub just

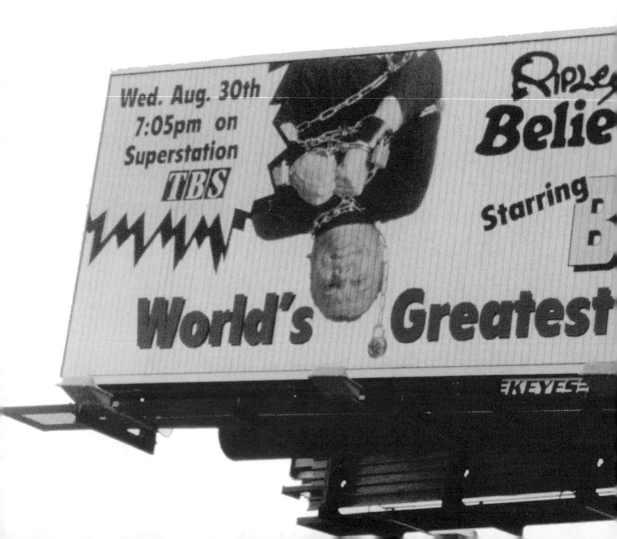

big enough for a 15-foot Burmese python. There was a part of me that wanted to leave the little guy there for the next pair of lovebirds who checked in, or to see the maid's face when she cleaned. I did put up the DO NOT DISTURB sign.

After dinner we returned to the room. Yes, the snake was still there. I hadn't given much thought to the actual escape, figuring it would be pretty simple. But my nephew Jimmy, who had accompanied Battson and me to Hollywood, asked the $64 question:

"Hey, Uncle Bill, have you ever gotten out of three straitjackets?"

"Well, what kind of a stupid question is that? Do you think I'd have accepted this gig if I had never gotten out of three straitjackets?"

"Yeah, I do, Uncle Bill." Battson agreed.

"You're right. We'd better start practicing."

> **"Well, what kind of a stupid question is that? Do you think I'd have accepted this gig if I had never gotten out of three straitjackets?"**

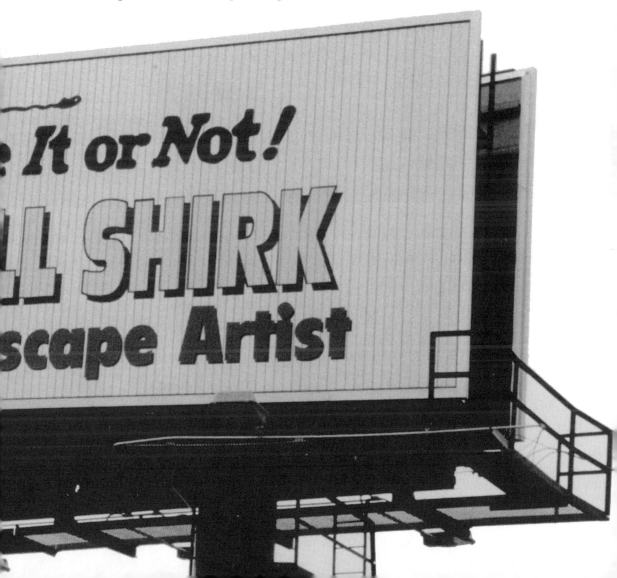

And practice we did. And guess what? I couldn't do it. I was trying a new method in which I immediately freed one arm under the jacket before they put the other jackets on. This allowed me to manipulate the snake in such a way that it would appear he was choking me, but even with the loose arm I couldn't get enough leverage to free myself from the other two jackets. This concerned me. I couldn't get out from the restraint in my hotel room standing up, with no snake. I'd be upside down in less than twenty-four hours. Uh-oh.

"Say, Uncle Bill, why don't you just go back to your old method? I bet that would work." Battson was just shaking his head and laughing.

I reverted to my old method and was out in forty seconds. Remember, this was three straitjackets. *Ripley's*, here we come.

The next morning the four of us (counting the snake) headed out. As we neared the Hollywood Hills, a breathtaking monastery came into sight. This was the location for the shooting of the *Ripley's* special. We drove the van through the gates and were in awe of the majestic marble and brick buildings.

> **This was no B-movie set (and I knew the makings of a B movie when I saw one). There must have been thirty crew people, six or eight cameras, tripods, cranes, and lights. Man, this was big time.**

This was no B-movie set (and I knew the makings of a B movie when I saw one). There must have been thirty crew people, six or eight cameras, tripods, cranes, and lights. Man, this was big time.

"But where are the other people?" I asked.

"You're it," said the producer. "It's all about you."

Truth is, there would be others on the show. Like a guy who'd lost the top of his head doing a motorcycle stunt; some nut who'd gone over a fourteen-story waterfall in a kayak and almost drowned; and a woman who'd died in a boat crash and was brought back to life.

Yes, they would all be on the show as well, but their video would be supplied to *Ripley's* by the participants, shot by friends or an independent film company. I was to be the main feature, and they wanted to film my escape themselves. I was a little nervous. Most of the other people in the show had been seriously hurt doing their stunt. Did they want me to be an exception, or part of an overall theme?

The show was a success. I appeared in a puff of smoke. Jimmy put me in the three straitjackets as a local police officer watched over the procedure. They hung me upside down; Battson brought out the 150-pound snake, wrapped him around me, and they hoisted me up 60 feet. The snake got an immediate hold around my throat, but I had developed a technique to prevent being strangled. By putting my chin flush against my chest, I protected my airflow even though it appeared as if the snake was choking me.

Great TV, though, and I enhanced the effect by holding my breath and making my eyes bulge out. The crew was really into it, but concerned I was having the life sucked out of me. One camera shot was right in my face. When I watched it on TV a month later, it even scared the heck out of me.

The escape was over. They brought me down. The producer was elated. He came over to congratulate me. *This was too much fun*, I thought to myself. Wait a second. Did I say *fun*? I had never felt that doing an escape had really been fun. There was always a motive, a reason to take such chances. But damn, this was fun.

Suddenly, I found myself saying to the producer: "Let's do it one more time."

The crew erupted in applause and laughter. I mean, who else would say that but crazy Bill Shirk? The crew loved me. The producer loved me. I was loving myself. We did it again. And it was fun again.

The night it aired, the *Ripley's* program was the number one cable show for that Wednesday night and the biggest audience *Ripley's* had ever had for one of their specials.

I was about as high as I had been in years. But things were going to get better, better than I ever dreamed they could get.

> **They hung me upside down; Battson brought out the 150-pound snake, wrapped him around me, and they hoisted me up 60 feet. The snake got an immediate hold around my throat, but I had developed a technique to prevent being strangled.**

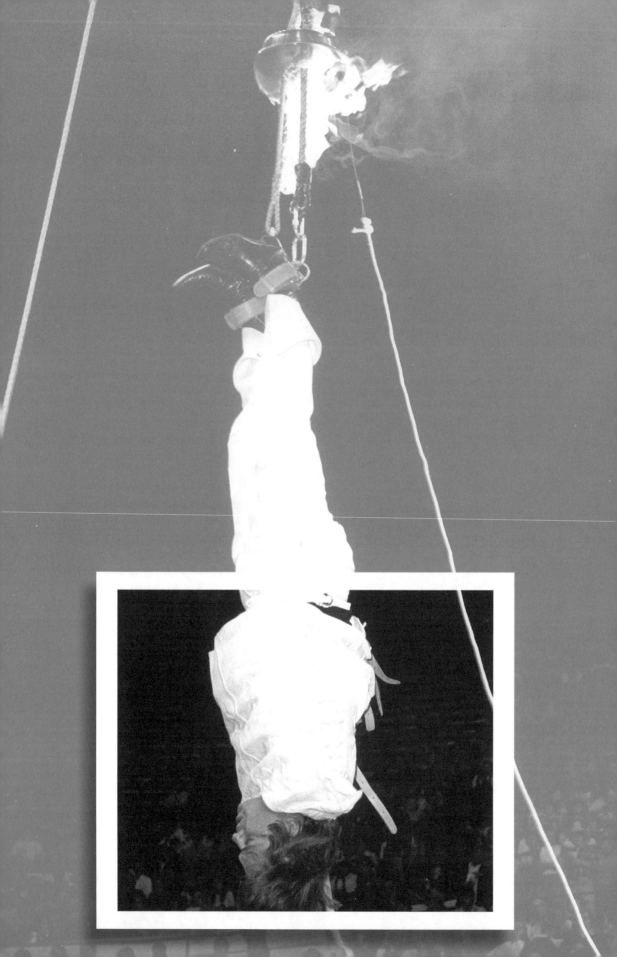

SHIRK.DOCumentary

IN MEDIA CIRCLES Bill Mays and I were known as Dollar Bill and Crazy Bill. Mays was the bank; I was the crank. Neither of us minded. Especially when in June 2000, Radio One—a huge, publicly traded, minority-owned company—offered Bill and me $40 million for our properties. One local radio mogul called it a financial Houdini. Now that's a compliment!

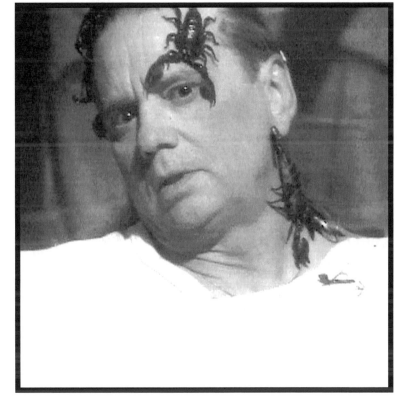

I don't mean to simplify months of negotiations, but this book is about escapes, not business deals. I will tell you this: That was the most ever paid for a group of low-powered radio and TV stations. Ever. Am I bragging? You betcha.

It was more money than I ever dreamed of having. I wrote my wife a check for a million bucks. After reading this book, you probably think she deserved more. I set up a trust fund for my daughter, Maxine. When I had a few moments, I sent the IRS enough to build new headquarters. And I built a pond. And next to it a multimillion-dollar estate.

Radio One wanted me to stay on and run the radio stations, which I did for a while, but I finally resigned and decided to stay home and enjoy myself. That novelty lasted about two weeks, at which point I was climbing the walls. Just the idea that there was no action to look forward to, no stunts, no escapes, no radio station to promote, was making me realize that I really was an adrenaline junkie—and one with a big ego. What a combination.

It was time to do a documentary of my life. Not like the movie, though. No goofy characters, bad acting, and making love from a chandelier. No, this would be a serious chronicling of all the stunts and escapes I had done, many of which I had on video but had never really taken the time to archive appropriately. It would also be a way of portraying my life in the context of Harry Houdini's. Houdini had been my mentor and hero, but in more than a few ways I had surpassed him. I wanted my daughter and grandkids someday to know that.

I chose Nineteenth Star to do the job, an Indianapolis company that had already produced several award-winning documentaries and was headed by Tom Cochrun, a friend and former television news anchor whose judgment I trusted. While I had never really bristled at the label *crazy*, I did feel that the documentary in some way needed to establish the seriousness of my pursuits and my commitment to the Houdini legacy.

As well as previously shot video, I decided to perform four stunts staged specifically for the documentary. The first was the simplest. I wanted to break my straitjacket record of 4.53 seconds that been in the 1979 edition of the *Guinness Book*. At this point Guinness had opted to play down escape records, but it mattered to me that I could say I had officially beaten my old time from twenty-five years earlier. I did break that record. Total time: 4.49 seconds.

The second escape was a bit more elaborate. I was chained and handcuffed, then placed in a bag with a 14-foot python, once again a reptilian associate of Larry Battson. In this escape it was important to get free of the restraints before the snake was introduced through the top of the bag. As before, we had allowed the snake to spend a few pleasant evenings with various Bill Shirk odors and bodily fluids so he'd feel like we were old friends.

When the snake entered headfirst (which is the preferred method, so as not to have him surprised by a human sharing his space), I grabbed him by the back of his neck and then wrapped him around me for effect. Minutes later I emerged

When the snake entered headfirst (which is the preferred method, so as not to have him surprised by a human sharing his space), I grabbed him by the back of his neck and then wrapped him around me for effect.

Things They Don't Teach You in *The Worst-Case Scenario Handbook*

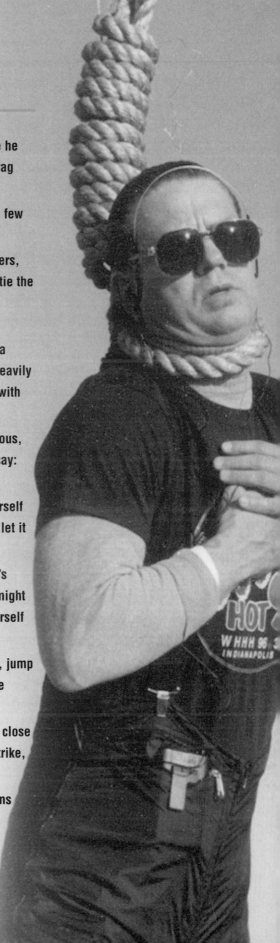

1. When sharing a coffin with a rattlesnake, be sure he slept on ice the night before. And treat him to a rag soaked with your urine. He'll never forget you.

2. If you plan on being thrown in jail, visit the jail a few days before and hide a key.

3. If you find yourself in an enclosed area with spiders, tarantulas, or scorpions, take off your pants and tie the critters up inside. Then try not to make a *whoop-whoop-whoop* noise like the Three Stooges.

4. If you plan to hang over a killer whale tank from a burning rope in ninety-degree heat, don't drink heavily the night before. Same advice if you plan to run with the bulls in Pamplona.

5. If you have to do something really, really dangerous, do it on April 1. Then you can fudge a little and say: "April fool!"

6. If you are being placed in a straitjacket, puff yourself up like a blowfish. When the jacket is tightened, let it all out. You'll have some wiggling room.

7. If you want a train to run over you, be sure there's enough room under the train. If there isn't, you might as well get hit head-on by the train and save yourself the trip down.

8. Whether you are going to hang from a helicopter, jump off a bridge, or just walk in a mall, wear sensible shoes.

9. If you find your head in a bag with a rattlesnake, close your eyes. This won't reduce the chances he'll strike, but at least you won't have to see yourself die.

10. If you want to buy three low-powered radio stations and a TV station for $4 million, be sure you can sell them for $40 million seven years later.

through the top of the bag free of the chains and handcuffs with the python around my neck and chest.

The third escape was a throwback to the head-in-the-bag-with-a-rattlesnake. As I mentioned in the previous chapter, Battson was out of congenial reptiles, but he did have one snake with a penchant for striking out at the first sight of a probe. After the initial hit, the snake seemed sated and returned to a kind of resting state. Incredibly, Battson saw an advantage in this predictable peculiarity.

"Bill, this is great. We'll take your ponytail and we'll redistribute your hair to the top of your head, then slather it with some hair gel so it hardens, and connect a tiny tube camera to it. When your head slides down into the bag, he'll take one strike at the camera, and we'll have some great video."

"You're crazier than I am," I told Battson. "Of course, I could top that by listening to you."

Truth is, I trusted Larry. I knew that his success was in part connected to mine. If anything happened to me, his snakes would be out of work. And Larry sure wouldn't do a stunt like this himself. He was scared to death of snakes. (That's not really true, but if he doesn't complain about my saying that, I'll know he didn't read this book.)

First I was tied in 25 feet of rope, then hung upside down from a block and tackle. My head was then placed in the bag where the snake had been lounging around for several hours. I heard the hissing and closed my eyes. I did not want a face-to-face with the rattler. As I worked to free myself from the rope, he struck at the camera on top of my head, resulting in a breathtaking shot, which, like the *Ripley's* video, still gives me the creeps every time I see it. Once the snake hit the camera, he calmed down as Battson predicted. I finished getting out of the rope in a matter of minutes and popped my head out of the bag. The Nineteenth Star crew was almost catatonic watching this. If you ever have an opportunity to buy my documentary, you must see this. Oh, what a

> **As I worked to free myself from the rope, he struck at the camera on top of my head, resulting in a breathtaking shot, which, like the *Ripley's* video, still gives me the creeps every time I see it.**

coincidence. Here's an opportunity: Go to my Web site, www.Billshirk.com.

In the final escape, I was placed in a Plexiglas coffin in double straitjackets with thirteen black widow scorpions and a bucket full of Amazonian cockroaches. Please remember that I had several million dollars in the bank and could have been smoking a $200 Cuban cigar on the balcony of a $2,000-a-day room in Maui. I just wasn't ready for that. Not yet.

The escape took longer than I had thought, almost fifteen minutes, during which time I feared that the scorpions would get into the straitjacket and sting me as I tried to escape the restraints. They had a different idea. Instead of hiding in my straitjacket, they decided to hold a tag-team match with the cockroaches on my face. After a few minutes of hissy fits, they called it quits. Thank goodness. They were tearing up the playing field.

I got the jackets off in about five minutes, then loosened the hinges on the inside of the coffin and essentially dismantled the box.

The documentary met and exceeded my expectations. And it led to an offer by the Travel Channel to use my seven-ton dirt-cement burial as part of a special about the Houdini Museum in Appleton, Wisconsin. Involved in the show were Lance Burton, probably the top magician in the world, and Sid Radner, a Houdini historian and writer. Burton, by the way, had done an escape on a roller coaster (see Five Great Escapes Someone Else Did) that I would consider one of five best ever performed.

I, of course, did the other four.

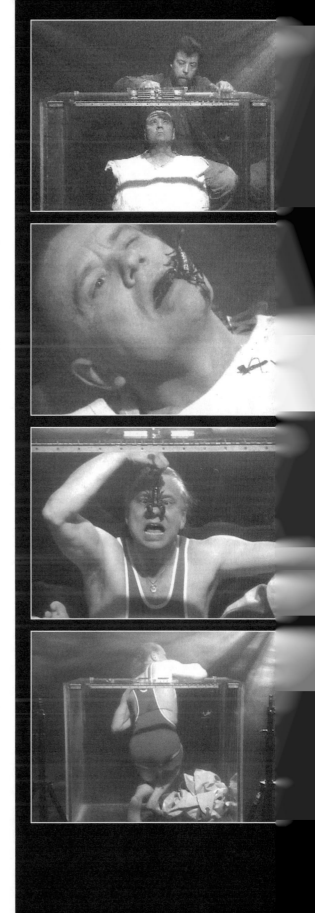

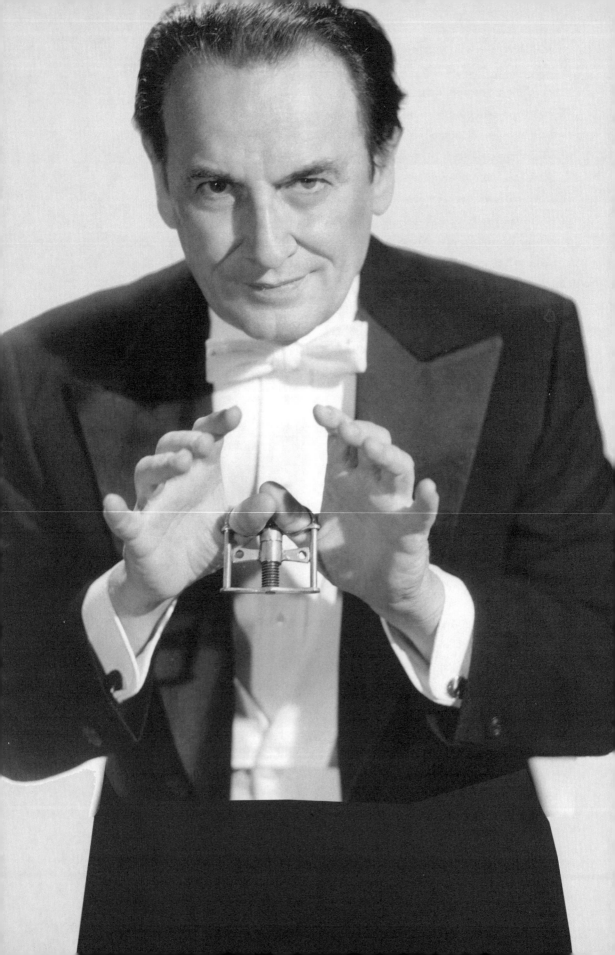

Five Great Escapes Someone Else Did

1. In the 1950s Milbourne Christopher caught a bullet (shot from a gun) in his mouth on national TV. This was *not* an illusion. He really did it.

2. In the mid-1990s, Lance Burton was handcuffed and chained to the track of a roller coaster, escaping just seconds before the out-of-control roller coaster would have cut him in two.

3. David Copperfield's upside-down straitjacket escape hanging from three burning ropes. This was a rip-off of my triple burning rope escape. My gear cost about fifty bucks. Copperfield's rigging for his national TV show cost $25,000. But I still loved it. In fact, I was flattered.

4. In the 1980s Dean Gunnarson, a Canadian escape artist, was handcuffed, chained, and put in a coffin. The coffin was lowered into an icy river. He was brought up fifteen minutes later and pronounced dead at the scene, still in the restraints. One hour later at the hospital, he was revived and brought back to life. While his intention was not to almost die, he did perform the ultimate escape by coming back from death, a feat even Houdini dreamed of doing.

5. As depicted in a 1953 movie, Tony Curtis, playing Houdini, was handcuffed and chained, put into a box, and lowered through a giant hole in the ice-covered Detroit River. The real Houdini once did jump into the Detroit River while handcuffed, but there was no ice. He also had a safety rope around his waist. But the myth surrounding this escape grew and the story got better and better, culminating in the movie scene described above. Houdini never set the record straight. Why would he? To this day, many believe that Houdini died doing this escape. He didn't. He died of appendicitis.

   This is quite possibly the world's most dangerous escape . . . that was never done. But I plan on doing it someday.

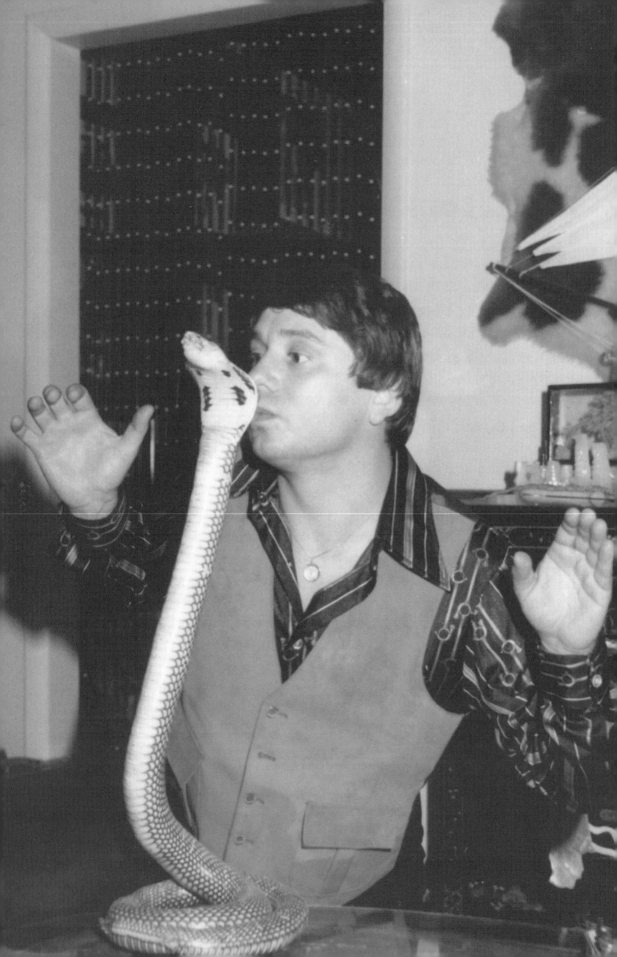

Epilogue

IN THE FALL OF 2002, I was asked to be part of a new book called *Indiana Curiosities*, a collection of oddball people and happenings in Indiana, published by The Globe Pequot Press. The author, Dick Wolfsie, is a local TV reporter, so it never dawned on me he was smart enough to write a book. But I liked his style and realized this was the guy to help me tell my story, the whole story. Everything.

Dick has the cushiest TV job in America. He goes out every morning and talks to people like me who have interesting offbeat jobs, or hobbies, or talents.

I wanted to give him something to do with all his free time so I asked him to help me write my memoirs.

I had always taken my escapes very seriously, but I knew that there was a funny side to all I had accomplished. Dick has helped communicate that. We spent many, many hours working together at my large, luxurious home. For a while I wondered if he was just casing the joint, a trick he would have learned from writing this book.

Everything you have read (or will read, if you skipped to the back page) is true. I have never previously divulged to the public the inside story of my mistakes or the secrets to my successes.

By now I have probably gone on to new escapes. I have always wanted to do the underwater box escape first performed by Harry Houdini more than fifty years ago, an escape that even freaked him out because of its connection with burial. That's why Houdini called it a box, not a casket. Some have almost died doing this one.

Then I'd like to perform the underwater burial—not just underwater, but under a frozen pond—an escape that has never been accomplished or even attempted. And I have a pond behind my house. What a coincidence.

So now that you've read the book, what do you think? Am I crazy? Not sure? Just remember one thing: If I were really crazy, I'd be dead.

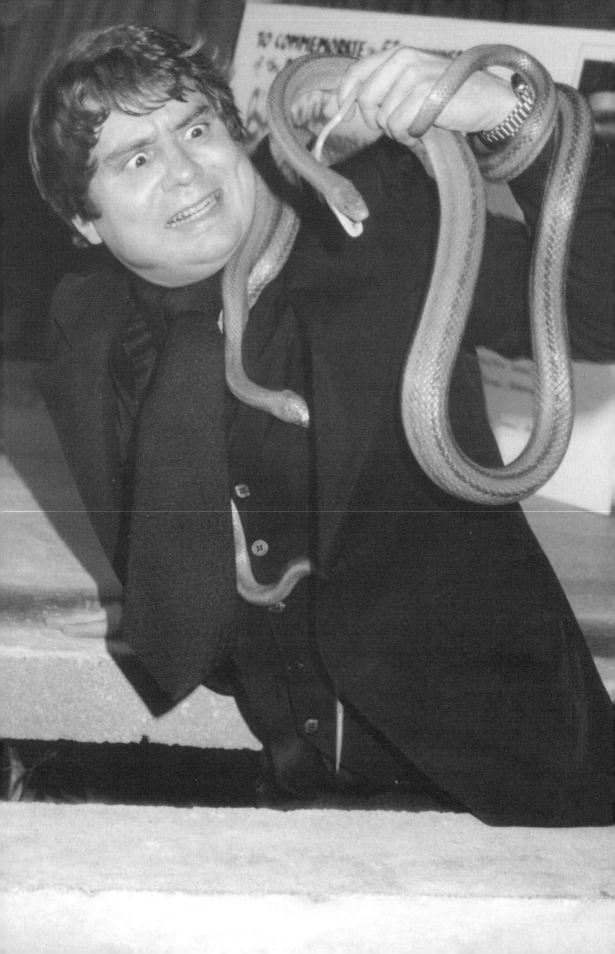

About the Authors

BILL SHIRK has been doing daring escapes for more than a quarter of a century. While some superlatives are subjective, the title World's Number One Escape Artist certainly can be applied to Bill Shirk, who over the past twenty-five years has held multiple records in escapology, most of which have been listed in the *Guinness Book of World Records*.

Over the past thirty years in Indianapolis, Bill Shirk has bought and sold a slew of radio and TV stations and confounded critics and skeptics alike by not only escaping bankruptcy (he can escape anything), but ultimately turning a handsome profit, as well.

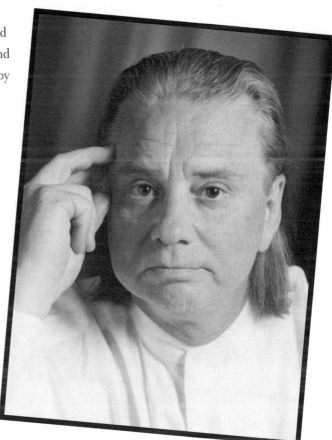

Now as co-owner of Hoosier broadcasting, Shirk oversees three virtual radio stations (if you don't know what "virtual radio" means, read the book) and spends time with his wife Liz and twelve-year-old daughter Maxine. They all live together in Zionsville, Indiana in a home that those pesky critics and skeptics said he'd never be able to afford.

DICK WOLFSIE has taught high school and college, hosted three TV talk shows and one radio show, and has written four books. Winner of two national entertainment awards, a regional Emmy, and a dozen local awards, he's interviewed more than 15,000 people and done more than 5,000 hours of live radio and television in Indiana alone.

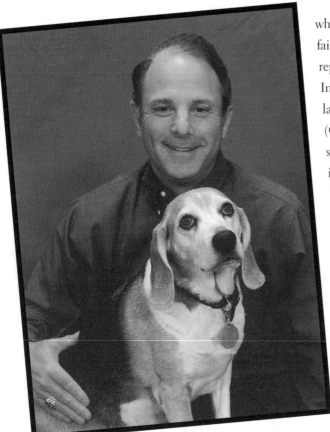

Dick has been accompanied everywhere he goes—including work—by his faithful beagle, Barney. He has been a reporter on WISH-TV Channel 8 in Indianapolis for the last ten years. His latest book is *Indiana Curiosities* (Globe Pequot, 2003). Dick is also a syndicated humor columnist appearing in newspapers throughout Indiana.

Dick lives in Indianapolis with his wife, Mary Ellen, and Brett, his son.